Joy at Birth

This book draws on a collection of stories of birth from mothers, birth partners, obstetricians and midwives that demonstrate joy at birth across professional groups and in different types of births and locations, with or without technological interventions.

To be at the birth of a baby is special, providing experiences that touch us in ways difficult to articulate. For most of us, parent, birth partner and healthcare provider, it is a precious time like no other. Following an historical and contextual survey of childbirth, which highlights myriad changing moods around birth, focus is drawn to contemporary lived experiences at birth. Using hermeneutic phenomenology inquiry, this book reveals something extraordinary in the everydayness of childbirth experiences that are often overlooked. Joy is shown as emerging within a special quality of time – named Kairos – a time in which spiritual and existential encounters bring remembrance of our creativity and shared natality. The inquiry shows all types of births, wherever they happen, whatever the outcomes, are always significant and profoundly meaningful.

It will be of great interest to midwives, and those working in and studying maternity, obstetrics and neonatology, as well as social and medical anthropology, sociology, cultural, organisational and clinical psychology, and spirituality.

Susan Crowther is a visiting professor of midwifery at Robert Gordon University, Aberdeen, Scotland, a freelance senior academic, researcher, author, editor, reviewer, and occasional locum rural caseload midwife residing in New Zealand.

Routledge Research in Nursing and Midwifery

For more information about this series, please visit: www.routledge.com/Routledge-Research-in-Nursing/book-series/RRIN

Joy at Birth

An Interpretive, Hermeneutic,
Phenomenological Inquiry

Susan Crowther

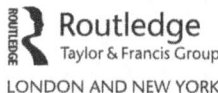
Routledge
Taylor & Francis Group

LONDON AND NEW YORK

First published 2020
by Routledge
2 Park Square, Milton Park, Abingdon, Oxon OX14 4RN

and by Routledge
52 Vanderbilt Avenue, New York, NY 10017

Routledge is an imprint of the Taylor & Francis Group, an informa business

First issued in paperback 2021

British Library Cataloguing-in-Publication Data
A catalogue record for this book is available from the British Library

Library of Congress Cataloguing-in-Publication Data
A catalogue record has been requested for this book

ISBN: 978-1-138-38915-1 (hbk)
ISBN: 978-1-03-208988-1 (pbk)
ISBN: 978-0-429-42414-4 (ebk)

Typeset in Times New Roman
by Wearset Ltd, Boldon, Tyne and Wear

Contents

Illustrations

About the author

Susan has worked in health care since 1983 and in the area of childbirth for over 26 years. Her interests extend to practice, education, and research into midwifery and maternity care provision. She has worked in many regions across the world as a midwife: UK, France, Russia, Armenia, Norgorno Karabagh, Malawi, Rwanda, Ghana, Burkino Faso, and long periods of time in New Zealand. Susan has worked in many ways, including practice as employed and self-employed caseload midwife, education as a senior lecturer, at strategic levels as a consultant midwife, and actively involved in research as professor of midwifery. Over this time and through these roles, she has maintained a keen interest in the spirituality of childbirth and the lived experiences of all those involved in childbirth, both professionally and personally. She regularly publishes in peer-reviewed international journals and has authored several chapters for textbooks. Susan engages with several peer review journals on their editorial boards and as a reviewer. She is an active member of the Research Standing Committee of the International Confederation of Midwives. Susan and co-editor, Dr Jenny Hall, published *Spirituality and Childbirth: meaning and care at the start of life* with Routledge in 2017. She authors a blog that explores continuity of carer practice in midwifery and spirituality in and around childbirth and is invited to deliver keynote lectures on a variety of topics including spirituality and childbirth and methodology focused seminars. Susan is interested in approaches to maternity that opens the vision for ongoing developments that incorporate physical, psychic, and spiritual dimensions to human experience through engagement with all stakeholders touched by childbirth, both medical and non-medical. She co-chairs the UK annual institute for Hermeneutic Phenomenology which provides research methodology courses and symposiums – a collaborative project between the University of Central Lancashire and Robert Gordon University. Currently, Susan is living back in New Zealand and working as a freelance senior academic and remains a visiting professor of midwifery at Robert Gordon University, Aberdeen, Scotland.

Acknowledgements

Projects such as this do not just appear without the contributions of many. Much gratitude to the participants who have shared their experiences that underpin this whole book. Without their stories this phenomenological inquiry would not have happened. Gratitude must go to Liz Smythe who is, at once, a thesis supervisor, a sounding board, friend, colleague, editor, and insightful ideas provider! Thank you, Liz, for proofreading parts of this book and offering your wisdom and the gift of your wonderful foreword. Thanks must also go to the reviewers of the original book proposal – I do not fully know who you all are, but thank you for giving me the go-ahead and giving constructive ideas which have helped shape the unfolding of this book. To the publishers and editor at Routledge. They have been supportive despite changes in staffing and have consistently encouraged me to keep going even when deadlines got pushed! To members of my New Zealand spiritual inquiry group who open me to myriad horizons of understanding about life's interconnected wholeness. Appreciation for Toby, my husband, who survived years of my midwifery on-calls, doing my PhD, and now writing this book. Partners of midwives are generally remarkable and mine is no exception. His patience is simply amazing and his capacity to gently remind me to 'get on with it' and ask, 'what do you need to get you into that office and typing?' There are so many others who have contributed to the thinking behind this project along the way – to you all, much gratitude.

Foreword

In her pre-academic life, Susan was an on-call midwife for many years. It is a life of getting up in the middle of the night when one is still tired from the last birth. It is seldom being able to commit to a social event knowing you could be called to a birth at any time. It is subjecting your husband to the uncertainty of never knowing when you will be home. It is travelling to the base hospital with a woman in the ambulance and after the birth finding oneself stranded. It is to carry the huge responsibility of care. It is personal sacrifice.

What is it that calls midwives to such service? Yes, they have a commitment to support women and their families in childbirth, but is that enough to accept such huge demands on your time and energy that impinge on your own wellbeing?

Yet, any midwife will tell you what an amazing privilege it is to be with a family when their new baby is born. There is 'something' that happens in that moment, something that lingers in the air, something that enlivens and inspires.

In this book, Susan takes on the impossible task of putting language to that 'something'. The stories take us back to a birth where the 'something' emerges from between the lines. Susan ponders on the glimpse, and unpacks the elusive meaning, gently wooing it into language.

Why does this book matter? In an age where technology so easily dominates, where staff privilege the mechanistic ways of the institution over what matters for those who give birth, where family retreat back into their shell to shield themselves from intimidation, that 'something' can so easily be lost. It can only be protected and preserved if we first remember what it is, and how much it matters.

Susan names the something as 'joy'. Such a short, simple word. Joy 'is'. Joy 'comes'. Joy is 'amazing'.

Read this book to embrace second-hand moments of joy. More importantly, read this book so you too will be inspired to join the movement intent of ensuring that every family has a space woven around them that enables joy to come, to flourish.

I suspect that when a baby is birthed into an ambience of joy, something deeply impactful is rooted for the rest of his/her life. There is no way we could ever prove such a thing. But imagine if it were true and you were part of the institutional care that brushed aside such 'soft' mandates of care. How unsafe could that be?

Susan is to be applauded for breaking the silence and for bringing the courageous voice of 'love' into an academic world more familiar with 'evidence' and 'outcomes'.

Let her take you on the journey. You will remember afresh what you already know.

Professor Liz Smythe
Auckland University of Technology
New Zealand
May 2019

Part I

An invitation into a clearing

A clearing is more than a space. It is where something has been cleared away. A clearing offers us an opening through which new horizons of understanding and insights can bubble up into thought through hitherto previously unknown pathways of thinking. A clearing is a space where we find ourselves and others emerging out of darkness, hiddenness, and covered-up-ness where what was invisible and obscured by shadow comes into the light. In this new light, we can now see the concealed and appreciate that which remains concealed. To find oneself in such a clearing is to be transformed and illuminated so that we can glimpse possibilities on our journey ahead.

As the philosopher Martin Heidegger reminds us:

> In the midst of beings as a whole an open place occurs. There is a clearing, a lighting.... Only this clearing grants and guarantees to us humans a passage to those beings that we ourselves are not, and access to the being that we ourselves are. Thanks to this clearing, beings are unconcealed ... yet a being can be concealed too, only with the sphere of what is lighted.
>
> (Heidegger, 1971/2001: 51–52)

Reference

Heidegger, M. (1971/2001). *Poetry, Language, Thought.* New York: HarperCollins.

1 Introduction

To be at the birth of a baby is special, an experience that often touches us in ways that are difficult to articulate. For most of us, parent, healthcare provider, or/and support person (accidental or planned), it is a precious experience like no other. However, there is an increasing secularisation and reliance on technology in contemporary maternity care, particularly in the western context. Amongst this growing dependence on technology there is a concern that something of significance at birth gets concealed and silenced. Technological birth, natural or normal birth, and holistic social models as opposed to medicalised models of care are well defined and extensively written about by their protagonists. Yet the experience of joy when a baby is born and how that is meaningful to those present has received little attention. This book turns our attention to this silence, returning our focus to experiences of being there at the moment of birth and the experience of joy.

Joy at birth is something that matters in ways not yet fully articulated or investigated. To be touched and affected by a mood (which I am naming 'joy' mindful of the limits of any one word) has both intrigued and invoked passion. Birth arouses the imagination. It is a mystery in which all of us have been involved (Forbes-Rogers, 1966). Birth has been seen as a rite of passage which has been identified as a re-enactment of the myth of the divine mother and child (Campanelli and Campanelli, 1998), a joyful occasion of great significance that is often experienced as a numinous occasion and "…the first act of magic" (Razak, 1990: 168).

Exactly how joy transcends the type, place, and who is present at birth remains elusive. Rhetorical debates continue in the literature and in practice. The social and medical sciences provide knowledge and expertise that assists in alleviating human suffering and minimising loss of life. Birth has a profound meaning beyond social, political, and cultural descriptions. There is something magical that inheres within the experience of being at birth that remains hidden yet embedded within the wholeness of the experience itself. In the process of a hermeneutic literature[1] review, I found little regarding the experiential and meaningful aspects of the moment when a baby is born (Crowther *et al.*, 2014). For me, this posed unresolved and unanswered existential questions about what birth 'is' and how 'it' is experienced and meaningfully interpreted.

This book contains the principal findings of my PhD hermeneutic phenomenology study as well as continuing research, writings, thinking, and ongoing interpretations of the phenomenon 'joy at birth'. In the PhD, stories of being at birth were collected from mothers, birth partners, obstetricians, and midwives in face-to-face interviews. These are the stories presented in this book. Joy at birth was experienced across professional groups and in different types of births and locations, with or without technological interventions. Through exploration of these experiences something extraordinary was revealed which is often ignored and overlooked beyond the activities that help ensure survival. In exploring this phenomenon through the words of those present at the time of birth, I sought to reveal some of the *felt* aspects that constitute the phenomenon of joy at birth. Thus, I began to question what was going on, I kept asking: What is the experience of 'joy' at the birth of a baby and how is this joy significant and meaningful? At the same time, I acknowledged that there was never going to be any fixed and complete answers to any phenomenon – what I have attempted to do in this work was gesture a direction of thinking and ongoing inquiry.

The key aims of this book are:

- Provide in-depth insights into the experience of joy at birth
- Invite thinking about 'how' we are and 'what' we do at birth

This introductory chapter poses the question: What is meant by and what is the meaning of joy and how does it affect childbirth? Whilst birth satisfaction is important, this chapter orientates the reader to experience(s) in, and around, birth. Same or different, meaningful experiences are not always happy or satisfactory experiences, and, in the same way, joyful experiences are not necessarily exuberant in their manifestation. Each chapter introduces stories of joy that reveal multiple meanings. In addition, each chapter links with previous and subsequent chapters, highlighting embodied, spatial, and relational meaning. As the chapters unfold, a coalescence of experiential qualities at birth reveal insights of a timeless moment – named Kairos at birth – involving numinous encounters and connections across generations and revealing an overwhelming joy at birth. Joy is revealed as a *felt sudden awakening* that gestures to what it means to be human. This is not to say that all births are straightforward. Even when such joy is seemingly hidden and covered over – such as, when there are poor outcomes – joy shows itself in the experience of being at birth through our care and concern.

How language itself can 'speak us' and how texts interact with me, the investigator, and you, the reader, through a 'fusion of horizons'[2] is central to hermeneutic writing which uses language to convey what is meant (Gadamer, 1960/1975). Words have different meanings for different people, at different times and in different places. Gadamer tells us that language is a way of being in the world because words describe experience. It is therefore important that the words 'mood' and 'joy' which are specific to this study have their meanings clarified from the beginning.

The word 'mood' was discovered prior to the word 'joy' during the research proposal stage. In conversations with my supervisors at the time, coupled with ongoing reading, I explored words such as 'presence', 'sacred' and 'spiritual' to see how close they came to the feeling of the phenomenon of interest. Eventually, the word 'mood' arose as the most suitable way of moving the study towards something tangible. The Heideggerian interpretation of attunement or mood was the closest to what I was 'feeling' and experiencing about the phenomenon. Heidegger interprets mood as a state-of-mind or our way of being disposed to the world. He states: "A mood assails us" implying it befalls us suddenly as we are "thrown into situations" (Heidegger, 1927/1962: 175). Discovering and learning about this Heideggerian notion of attunement or mood was a eureka moment and provided a way forward into my inquiry. More about this notion will be explored in the following chapter.

Joy is a word that conjures many unique interpretations: great delight or happiness caused by something exceptionally good or satisfying; it can be a keen pleasure; elation, delight, something greatly valued or appreciated, an expression or display of glad feeling, a state of happiness, felicity, and cherished contentment (Harrison, 2010; Parse, 1997). One can feel joy; be glad and rejoice. A father expresses strong feelings at the birth of his daughter in an online blog: "... looking at her, I felt nothing but pure excitement and love for her, an explosion of joy; caused by a little girl in a bundle of blankets. Clearly anyone could have figured out why they call babies 'bundles of joy'" (Joe, 2011). This father's joy is experienced as a powerful and elevated emotion; a feeling that is something more than peace, more than delight; something akin to ecstasy.

Joy can be mixed with other powerful feelings (Harrison, 2010; Parse, 1997; Pilkington, 2006). For example, in Thompson's (2010) hermeneutic study, mothers' lived-experience following traumatic birth moments of expanded consciousness or apotheosis were revealed as transformative. These elevated divine states provided feelings and a sense of knowing about wholeness and connectedness. Joy does not have to be a state of effusive excitement, yet it brings a sense of peace and hope that is connecting, all-consuming, and holds potential for new understandings.

An ontological inquiry

Hermeneutic phenomenology is an ontological inquiry. It does not seek to construct labels of the phenomenon – thus contributing to a discourse – but rather reveal the 'Being'[3] of phenomenon surfacing hidden and unnoticed layers of meaning. In addition, ontological differs from an ontical focus. An ontological focused inquiry is about the Being of entities (beings) as opposed to the attributes of a being. In identifying attributes, we are speaking of entities and not the Being of those entities. In other words, ontological inquiry relates to the Being of objects, the existential meanings of objects. Let me illustrate further to clarify. If I take a professional midwife as an object in my world of research, I can determine what the attributes and qualities of that role are and arrive at some kind of fixed essential descriptive parts that make up the professional midwife. This is an ontic research exercise. Now, if I focus on what it is to Be a professional midwife, with its essential descriptive parts, my inquiry turns to an ontological inquiry drawing attention to the meaning, collective understanding, and interconnected relationship to the world in which this object (professional midwife) exists.

Introduction of these complex notions early on in this book allows you to become aware that the focus is not on measurable, material or physical phenomena, such as the physiology of joy and hormonal changes, the science of oxytocin or emotional psychometric scores. Rather, this book draws us towards an ontological focus. By employing the Heideggerian notion of a human being (Dasein), an ontological focus is sketched out that draws our focus to the everyday taken-for-granted ways of being at birth. This focus illuminates shared themes within our humanness at birth that unite us in our experiences of Being-there-at-birth rather than a focus on specific cultural, traditional, and medical practices.

It has been argued that this approach is suited to examination of experiences in and around childbirth and midwifery due to the contextual relational quality of childbirth phenomena (Bergum and Van Der Zalm, 2007; Miles *et al.*, 2013; Thomson *et al.*, 2011). Comprehensive understanding of childbirth requires a phenomenological view of health care that is not solely based on a Cartesian metaphysical approach that objectifies and reduces experiences to merely ontic concerns leaving existential meanings hidden.

The examination of joy at birth uncovers profound existential meanings that will provoke the reader to think beyond their own horizons of understanding and how contemporary maternity care is organised opening the possibility to think anew about birth and remind us that we are not only mortal beings but are primarily natal beings. This shared natality – a term used by Hannah Arendt – gestures to our creative possibilities that inhere at each birth beckoning us to (re)examine what and how we act, think, and care at each birth.

What do I bring?

My pre-understandings (what I bring) are an essential part of this inquiry. It is therefore important to highlight when I am speaking, therefore, the pronouns 'I' and 'my' are used to achieve this clarity. 'I' am part of the interpretative process and hence work in a dialectical[4] way with the data, my professional discourses, and the world of research throughout this inquiry.

I have practised in health care for 30 years; the majority of these within midwifery (practice, education, leadership, and research roles). With a keen interest in self-development, spirituality, and concepts related to holism that incorporate mind-body-spirit interconnectedness, I am intrigued by the emotional, feeling, and spiritual dimensions of human experience. I am not the person I was before becoming a midwife. Frequent exposure to this intense 'specialness' is a catalyst for inward change that appears to generate a passion in me.

The possibility of every birth being significant and joyous inspires me in ways that I am unable to articulate. I maintain that birthing practices have become increasingly secular and practical, particularly within the western medical reductionist paradigm that currently informs maternity care. The mention of mood of joy at birth is conspicuously absent in daily maternity practice. I argue that it is experienced but frequently passed by. Busy modern maternity care can be likened to walking with a friend in a flower garden talking through myriad concerns. We reach the end of the walk and have not turned to the roses and taken in their simple but intoxicating fragrance; we seem to have passed by an aesthetic opportunity.

I am therefore concerned that we are missing essential aspects of meaning that are always inherent during the time of birth. Contemporary birth technologies appear to be creating a framework which is self-perpetuating, obscuring the mystery of what birth 'is' by reducing it to aspects that are visible and measurable. I would argue that the distinctive vocabulary or language now dominating births are the discourses of risk aversion and medicalisation. As a consequence, emotional and spiritual aspects at the moment of birth have scarcely been researched and given little emphasis in modern maternity care provision. Yet evidence is emerging that unmet emotional needs can disrupt human physiology with adverse consequences for biological systems and relationships with others (Schulkin *et al.*, 2005). Research suggests that failing to understand physiological and emotional interactions is detrimental (Dixon *et al.*, 2013). Thankfully, current global research guidance and research priorities for maternity care are beginning to refocus on outcomes that aid women, families, and infants to thrive and reach their full potential not only survive birth (Downe *et al.*, 2018; WHO, 2018). However, there is still a need to explore existential, emotional, spiritual, and psychological outcomes of joyless birth experiences because we still do not know what the consequences are long term for all involved (Crowther *et al.*, 2019). I contend that there is a need to explore and clearly articulate the hidden yet significant experiential aspects of birth beyond the type, place, and outcome of birth alone.

Discordant voices and myriad discourses have produced a range of metanarratives surrounding childbirth. Appearing as dichotomous approaches to modern childbirth practices they conceal the essence of the birth experience. Yet as Tannen (1998) argues, this is a false dichotomy and a product of a society that thrives on arguments and wanting to win a position. It infers that there are rigidly marked partitions in these discordant voices and little recognition of a middle ground within which common meanings and significance can begin to be understood. It would appear that the world of birth is split into parts, all claiming validity and authority. We now dwell in a world with multiple horizons of understandings concerning birth that have difficulty fusing into something extraordinary. Disappointingly, these horizons often seem to remain far apart leaving us bereft of the possibility of a renewed vision for twenty-first century childbirth.

I would contend that this dichotomy is not jointly exhaustive. Everything that 'is' birth belongs to all perspectives and approaches. They cannot be mutually exclusive of each other. For example, at a highly technological birth there is still the possibility of a 'special' feeling just as there may be in a homebirth situation. There is no evidence to support that certain births are more joyful and special than others; this has certainly not been my professional experience. It is plausible, however, that some highly technologically focused births are less joyful in those immediate moments as other concerns take priority. In both situations a baby is born and is equally significant.

It is possible that the quality of personal relationships – and even society in general – would benefit from more positively attuned and meaningful birth experiences. It has been understood for some time that formative moments at birth are crucial for babies and parents, establishing patterns of intimacy and later ability to socialise (Winnicott, 1960; Kennell and Klaus, 1998; APPPH, 2013). This again points to something significant at birth. I am reminded of a colleague's comment: "I work on world peace one birth at a time" and another from a previous client: "if only the world remembered those moments at birth the world would be a better place". Fuller understanding of the moment of birth and its acknowledgement as significant and meaningful may indeed have important consequences yet unknown.

As a corollary of this incongruence in the birthing world there is growing concern amongst midwifery researchers that belief in women's ability to birth physiologically is being questioned. This is accompanied by fear that something of experiential significance is being lost in the pursuit of using technology (Fenwick *et al.*, 2010; McAra-Couper *et al.*, 2012). Perhaps there is something of experiential importance being lost in the face of 'technolust'.[5] The increasingly technological nature of contemporary westernised childbirth may not be without consequences. The meaning and significance of birth to families and those that support them through the childbirth experience in a technological atmosphere may be silencing something of significance and burying layers of meaning. Perhaps the increasing reliance and presence of technology at the birth of a baby undermines the fundamental essence of the experience and meaning of joy at birth.

Many researchers concerned about contemporary birthing practices have attempted to unravel the implications technological childbirth practices for babies, women and their families and communities, enquiring into woman-centred holistic practices that facilitate gentler, physiological, and empowering care whilst remaining safe. This is challenging because safety means different things to different people (Smythe, 2010). For example, women generally prioritise emerging unharmed and with a healthy baby but also seek peak and meaningful experience as central to the birth itself (Thomson, 2010; Parratt, 2010). Some women actively seek technology to make themselves feel safer (McAra-Couper *et al.*, 2012; Fenwick *et al.*, 2010), choose out of hospital births (Grigg *et al.*, 2015; Walsh, 2006; Edwards, 2013) whilst others choose to birth outside the local maternity systems and freebirth (out of hospital without midwifery or medical assistance) as this makes them feel safer (Holten and de Miranda, 2016; Plested and Kirkham, 2016).

In my experience, birthing women and those attending them have a need for physical safety but also to experience birth in some way as self-actualising (Maslow, 1964). The notion of ideal joyful birth implies an experience of self-actualisation[6] and/or peak experience connected to a meaning central to birth itself which provides a sense of fulfilment and purpose. For example, birth, as rite of passage, has been described as a powerful self-actualising experience manifesting an array of deepening insights (Cheyney, 2011; Lokugamage, 2011). Maslow (1964)[7] coined the term 'peak experience' to describe moments of joy in everyday experience making the distinction that they do not have a lineal progression as does the movement to self-actualisation. This is a key distinction. Peak experiences appear to catapult one into different awareness with new understandings recognisable to self and others. The experience of being at birth is more than about being safe; it is experientially meaningful.

The focus on safety is often born out of attuning to fear in and around birth that leads to an increase in risk averse behaviours resulting in overzealous use in some childbirth technologies. For example, the use of admission CTG monitoring on women admitted in early labour who have no 'risk' factors – despite extensive research to the contrary – in order to mitigate unease and improve safety. Yet there are glimpses of spiritual experiences in the literature that speak of these more existential qualities.

The concepts of spirituality and sacredness in childbirth are beginning to be explored more than in previous decades. Some authors have surmised that birth for some midwives, women, and medics evokes spiritual experiences (Doherty, 2010; Lahood, 2007; Lokugamage, 2011; Barrett, 2017). Spiritual and joyous experiences are personal and often occur in unexpected and surprising ways; what is unclear is if spiritual and existential experiences around birth lead to births that are satisfying. Satisfaction with birth studies have become more popular (Britton, 2012; Martin and Fleming, 2011; Sawyer *et al.*, 2013) yet they often do not focus on meaning and do not consider everyone present when a baby is born. The moments when a baby is born have often been named as spiritual (Gaskin, 1977; Crowther, 2019; Wojtkowiak and Crowther, 2018; Hennessey and Davis-Floyd, 2018). If spirituality involves a quest for the purpose in life and meaning to the project of living, then birth can be interpreted as the start of an on-going journey for family and community. Such potent experiences confront those at birth with something profoundly meaningful yet what that 'is' is often left unspoken. Unpacking the ineffable is not amenable to measurement, conventional scientific scrutiny or readily accessible through words.

Non-biological or non-rational experiences could be interpreted as instances of 'Being' or existence prior to thoughts that are pre-reflective. This 'in the moment experience' is an embodied knowledge or knowing that is not possible to conceptualise (Merleau-Ponty, 1962/2002). Moving beyond theories and concepts, rules and protocols is what captured my attention at the start of this inquiry. I felt there was so much more going on at birth than had been explicated through the myriad ontic concerns.

Many researchers continue to pursue ontic (material) lines of inquiry pertaining to childbirth (e.g. Church, 2016; Edwards *et al.*, 2018). I have no wish to further dichotomise thinking around birth and be disparaging about the ontic 'beings and entities' around birth, for these concerns are important and often prevent poor outcomes, but they do not fully illuminate the ontological qualities of that world. I suspect there are many factors influencing the birthing process beyond those recognised by the current bio-medical model and institutional organisation of maternity care. There is a need to explore the myriad meanings within the socio-cultural, historical, and linguistic contexts of those experiencing birth to reach deeper understanding. Birth holds differing meanings in different cultures and is interpreted according to different ethnic cosmologies. The affect or mood of birth holds sway in powerful ways over us.

Could the moment of joy at birth point to sacred significance and spiritual meanings that have been forgotten? I believe that joy at birth harbours rich meaning about our being there at birth; a phenomenon worthy of study and our collective thinking. Being personally drawn to discovering the meaning of joy at birth has significantly influenced this line of inquiry. From the genesis of the idea, there has been a consistent call.

> To hear a call is to be attuned to the always-there excitement, passion, or concern. If the idea leads only to thoughts of practicalities, or generates a yawn, then it is merely an idea, not a call.
>
> (Smythe, 2005: 232)

Responding to this call has never generated a yawn or desire to fix things. The call attuned me fully to a sense of wonder and spoke to who I am. Instead of attempting to explore the phenomenon without addressing my self-knowing and pre-understandings, I sought continually to make them visible and show how they have influenced my interpretations. Tina Koch (1996) refers to this as 'reflexivity' or the reciprocal relationship between the researcher and the subject of the research. I explicate this further in the next chapter.

The purpose of this inquiry was to bring the phenomenon 'joy at birth' to a 'feeling', to more fully articulate feeling aspects of the birthing phenomenon so that those gathered at birth recognise and acknowledge the specialness of the experience. I believe that mothers and those assisting them will benefit from understanding the significance and meaning of this 'joy'; an attuned joy that assails us, a feeling that allows for the experience of something deep and pro-found not often spoken about in the world of twenty-first century western birth. By bringing this phenomenon to light the less visible meanings of birth are named and illuminated. It is not the intention of this book to assume that that twenty-first century westernised childbirth practices are problematic, privative, or unwarranted, but rather to show how such approaches can conceal something significant and deeply meaningful. The chapters to follow do not seek to reveal an ultimate unmoving truth or theory, but to reveal, through existential interpre-tation, the phenomenon 'joy at birth' bringing it to 'feeling' and surfacing pos-sible hidden meanings.

Research design

To do this work was about choosing a path of meaning. A methodology that allowed for openness to new meanings. By drawing attention to the lived-experiences of those at birth, unspoken and unseen meanings could be foregrounded that would have otherwise remained concealed if examined through the lens of scientism. Thus, hermeneutic phenomenology was selected as a methodology and is elaborated fully in the following chapter. I now offer a brief summary of the research design or method, i.e. the nuts and bolts of what I did; the ontic elements of the inquiry.

Interview data was collected, following appropriate ethical approval, from 14 participants (4 mothers, 4 midwives, 3 obstetricians and 3 birth partners including a grandmother) via recorded and transcribed interviews. The participants were recruited by purposeful sampling and snowballing by word of mouth including professional networks within New Zealand. They were chosen for their experience of the phenomenon and interest in the study topic. A variety of perspectives in the study emerged until there was a sense of sufficiency in terms of variation of meaning. The aim was not to produce generalizable results but to direct questioning towards their experience of joy (or not) at birth and how that experience was meaningful. The quality of this inquiry was not dependent on demographic diversity as my purpose was not to compare difference but rather to invite other voices to merging conversations. It could be argued that different stake holders would have other crucial perspectives, but I realised that phenomenological research was never going to 'get it all' and never have it entirely 'wrapped up'. I considered the data to be sufficient when interpretations were both explicit and visible and fewer fresh insights were surfacing. This was never aiming for saturation but a point where more interviews and their resultant narratives became seemingly redundant.

A full detailed description of the research design, including ethics approval, recruitment, interview process, and data analysis can be found in the original thesis that is open access online.[8] The interviews took place over an eight-month period in the Auckland and Northland regions of New Zealand. Participants were encouraged to talk about any 'joy' experienced at birth through the narrating of their birth stories. The interview was undertaken in conversational style and encouraged the telling of detailed accounts of personal experience. Open ended questions were used to delve deeper for rich descriptions of experience. It was essential that detailed, rich, and nuanced descriptions of the lived-experience of joy at birth (or no joy) were captured in the participants' everyday language. Participants also lent me books, DVDs, recommended articles, shared poetry, and showed photographs revealing more than the dialogue of interviews and contributed to my thinking.

Stories were lifted from often brute everyday parlance of the raw data transcripts and 'polished'. Stories were often re-crafted in the writing and re-writing process as analysis deepened. More details about the process of crafting stories and data analysis have been published elsewhere (Crowther, 2016). Neither paraphrases nor verbatim quotes are used in the findings' chapters but parts or whole of these crafted and re-crafted stories powerfully brought the phenomenon to light and penetrated into layers of meaning. The crafted stories were returned to the participants to ensure they remained close to their detailed, described experience. This provided opportunity for clarification and for participants to request deletion of any part they did not want included in the study.

Like Caelli's (2001) experience of returning crafted stories to participants, several of the participants in this study were moved by their crafted stories. The final crafted stories were then used for interpretive analysis and are the stories presented in this book.

The interpretation of meaning from the stories sought to discern the significance of 'joy' at birth by surfacing meanings that have often remained unspoken. These narratives joined with my own experiences and thinking and a concurrent hermeneutic literature review of the literature – by combining all these threads of understanding in a fusion of horizons an illuminated, renewed appreciation came to light.

The iterative process of hermeneutic analysis can be disconcerting and challenging for the novice researcher and reader. I was constantly attentive to the tendency to drift towards psychological explanations (ontic entities) that depart from philosophical hermeneutic inquiry. Gadamer (2008/1967) explains how philosophical hermeneutics is a process of 'reading out' of texts not reading something into them. This was an iterative process of moving back and forth between the parts [interviews] and the whole [emerging analysis]. Each story had something to contribute to unveiling the phenomenon. I describe this process here in a three-level lineal way when, in fact, it was rather messy!

- Level one analysis began with crafting stories from verbatim data and describing what was in the data I had gathered. Then I took a hermeneutic (interpretive) move in the following ways.
- Level two analysis involved reading and re-reading the crafted stories to develop meanings from the data. At the same time, I needed to foreground my own pre-understandings to the interpretive process in an ongoing reflexive move. This stage was concerned with bringing out what was there in the text, between the lines, under and within the words used whilst acknowledging what I brought to the analysis. Tentative connections with philosophical writings and professional literature were introduced too. My reflexive stance and growing appreciation of the philosophical literature helped draw meaning from the stories whilst keeping the research question in front of me at all times. The inquiry was a journey of thinking and I remained always thinking in the working of the inquiry, as Heidegger states: "We never come to thoughts. They come to us" (Heidegger, 1971/2001: 6). As ontological patterns and qualities (often called themes in other qualitative methodologies) revealed themselves, they were noted.
- Level three analysis involved revisiting all level one and two interpretations, the literature, philosophical underpinnings, my field notes, and my pre-understandings. Other influences came into play such as conference presentations and the resultant conversations that arose. It was through the blending of stories and these multiple influences that an evolving fusion of horizons occurred. Insights and themes began to arise disclosing a commonality in the lived-experience of the phenomenon. This was a dwelling and bringing all together that evolved organically from the previous level of analysis. There was not a moment in clock time in which this level began to

be enacted; it came upon me as I found myself amidst and attuned to the interpretive process. Level two analyses were essentially about a deepening of understanding through reading, thinking, writing, re-reading, and re-writing. During this level of analysis, I delved deeper into the existential meanings being surfaced. In the thesis itself I describe two levels yet as my understanding developed post PhD, I started to see that there was a movement in which further interpretive leaps occurred during my reading of philosophical texts. For example, I spent a month researching the Heideggerian notion of attunement from multiple sources to help me better understand what I was 'seeing' in the data. Subsequent 'themes' were named in order to report them. This enabled me to comprehend more clearly what I was seeing whilst remaining elusive. To name something makes it easier to articulate, explore, and describe but it can also stop further thinking so a balance is always needed between what is reported and knowing that any insights from analysis that lead to the naming and reporting of 'themes' may change, however plausible they seem at the time.

Hermeneutic science is often subject to constraints and criticism because it does not have one clear approach to methodology and research design, thus it appears overly subjective (Paley, 2016). Hermeneutic phenomenology is an emerging iterative process and has no specific method. As Max van Manen says, "[a] phenomenological method cannot be fitted to a rule book, an interpretive schema, a set of steps, or a systematic set of procedures" (2014: 29). It is a journey of thinking and interpretation without recourse to creating fixed findings. The three levels of analysis emerged as a consequence of doing interpretive analysis; they were not the starting point. Each person starting a journey into hermeneutic phenomenology will find their own way. These possible three levels have subsequently been further explicated in a future publication (author – forthcoming).

Engaging with phenomena whilst remaining open to possibilities is central to this method and is its strength. Not settling for mere exploratory descriptions but surfacing interpretive meanings from context and content of lived-experience is an important tenet of realising the method. In other words, the trustworthiness of this methodology lies in its plasticity to method and explicit acknowledgement that the meanings of the experience within participants' stories intersect with those of the researcher (in this case me). The goal in this research was to bring these two meanings together in a fusion of horizons.

Introducing the participants

I now introduce the participants who gifted their stories for this inquiry. Women and/or partners who were experiencing some degree of depression following birth and practitioners involved in complaint proceedings were excluded. Midwifery students as well as anyone under my professional midwifery care during or prior to this study were also excluded. These exclusions were pragmatic and primarily for ethical reasons and in no way intends to undervalue the voices of those who did not share their experiences.

The women

- **Pat** – First time mother who planned and had homebirth. Caucasian.
- **Amy** – First time mother who wished for a homebirth but transferred to hospital and had a forceps birth. Caucasian.
- **Cathy** – First time mother who planned low intervention hospital birth but had induction of labour. Caucasian.
- **Laura** – Mother of two children. Both hospital births, one at 32 weeks gestation. Māori.

The birth partners

- **Tui** – Grandmother attending as birth partner for family and friends for 25 years. Community and hospital. Māori.
- **Karl** – Father of two. Present at both their homebirths, interviewed with his partner Pat. Caucasian.
- **John** – First time father. Present at hospital birth, interviewed with his partner Cathy. Māori.

The midwives

- **Diane** – Self-employed midwife over ten years; urban area. Also, midwife educator. Mother. Caucasian.
- **Simone** – Self-employed midwife over ten years; semi-rural areas. Mother. Worked in community and tertiary hospital settings both in the UK and NZ. Caucasian.
- **Marie** – Self-employed midwife over 20 years; urban-rural areas. Childfree. Caucasian.
- **Anahera** – Self-employed midwife over ten years; urban practice. Mother. Māori.

The obstetricians

- **Brenda** – Junior obstetrician. Childfree. Caucasian.
- **Carol** – Senior obstetrician worked both in NZ and overseas. Mother. Caucasian.
- **Steve** – Senior obstetrician working in both private and public services. Father. Caucasian.

You will be learning more contextual information about these participants through their narratives and the interpretive analysis in Chapters 4–7.

Full ethics approval was granted at the time of the study (see note viii below) and all participants gave permission for their stories to be used in publications following the PhD. All stories have been anonymised by change of names to pseudonyms, place names have been deleted and any other identifying information removed. All participants were provided with an opportunity to delete or change content in their data prior to final interpretive analysis.

The method of this study was a midwifing of understanding that facilitated remembrance of something hidden and/or forgotten in shadow. Yet I was aware that not all aspects of the phenomenon can be grasped as there is always something more than the "sum of specific incidents" (Dinkins, 2005: 118). I could have interviewed 100 more participants and still some of what the phenomenon 'is' would remain hidden from view. Something always remains in shadow; there is always more to discover.

This study is my unique interpretation of the interview data and contextually relevant literature mediated by my pre-understandings. This is congruent with the hermeneutic paradigm that holds no final proclamation. There was no uncontaminated place to be and no one interpretation is correct; the most plausible interpretations have been communicated. This book represents trustworthy phenomenological experiential data and rigorous interpretive analysis using established philosophical underpinnings to ensure congruence of interpretive insights.

Structure of the book

Reviewers of the book proposal asked, '*How is this book different to the PhD?*' This is my response. Although my original PhD study is available online, this book updates and brings an entirely different structure to the thesis, making the central messages more accessible to the reader not versed in the academic and health professional world or research methodologies. The material presented, however, will be useful to researchers – novice and experienced – who are new to this way of inquiry. In addition, this book draws upon my ongoing thinking, ideas, and ongoing related projects. The original PhD thesis, albeit having an international appeal in terms of focus, was conducted in the New Zealand context. As such many of the historical and contextual chapters are predominately New Zealand focused. Chapter 3 is thus a revised context and historical chapter to situate the study globally.

The structure and order of the thesis has also been changed to improve readability. For example, the literature review as a separate chapter has been removed and relevant literature added when pertinent to the context of each chapter. The full hermeneutic literature review has also been published separately (Crowther *et al.*, 2014). This book is divided into three sections.

Section one is about setting the scene and is focused on providing the philosophical underpinnings and historical context. Chapter 2 – the philosophical underpinnings – is key to appreciating the interpretive findings that follow. However, care is taken in this chapter to avoid terminology that could confuse the reader new to hermeneutic (interpretive) phenomenology. Some philosophical notions require specific words to describe them that are not in everyday spoken language use; in such cases, practical examples from everyday life will be used to illustrate their meaning. Chapter 3 examines the historical and contemporary context of the phenomenon.

The second section made up of four chapters is concerned with showing the phenomenon. The crafted stories used in Chapters 4–7 are from the PhD data set. Not all the stories were used in the final PhD and some stories are presented for the first time in these chapters to illustrate ongoing interpretive analysis and insights. The language in the final chapter in this section evolves into a more mantic style, conveying unspoken meanings that resisted being named. In this chapter poetic prose is employed as an invitation to join in a journey of thinking and enter a clearing in which concerns about birth can be pondered in new existential and ontological ways invoking new possibilities.

The third section is 'New Horizons' and presents ongoing thinking and new insights since completion of the PhD. This includes further developed interpretation of the notion Kairos time at birth and our shared natality. This final section also introduces and describes a more developed 'ecology of birth' first suggested in my previous edited book *Childbirth and Spirituality: Meaning and Care at the Start of Life* (Crowther and Hall, 2017). Finally, an epilogue provides a personal account of how doing this hermeneutic phenomenological inquiry has transformed me.

The next chapter returns to the philosophical underpinnings providing congruence with how and what made the inquiry hold together. Of course, if philosophy is not your 'thing' jump straight into the stories of Chapters 4–7 and enjoy.

Notes

1 A hermeneutic literature review differs from traditional ways of reviewing the literature. To review using a hermeneutic lens is not about predicting or providing final definitions through pooling, assembling, summarising findings, critiquing the analyses, or defining themes that lead to a theory or hypothesis. Rather, it is about how one is attuned and engaged philosophically with the literature. To review hermeneutically is to question, remaining engaged and staying open to the possibilities of what could be revealed. In this way questions and answers became a dialectical play and the literature is questioned in a particular fashion. Attuning questioning in this way deepens understanding, clarifying and refining the reviewer's focus. For insight into this way of reviewing the literature, see Smythe, E. and Spence, D. (2012). Re-viewing literature in hermeneutic research. *International Journal of Qualitative Methods*, 11, pp. 12–25.

2 Fusion of horizons: Gadamer talks of a 'horizon' as a way to conceptualise understanding. For example, your horizon is as far as you can see or understand childbirth from your own perspective. You have a horizon of understanding and so do I (the author of this book). I write this book with a horizon and you begin to read this book and encounter its contents with your own horizon. Gadamer explains that:

> the concept of horizon suggests itself because it expresses the superior breadth of vision that the person who is trying to understand must have. To acquire a horizon means that one learns to look beyond what is close at hand – not in order to look away from it but to see it better.

Thus, our understanding expands and changes when our present horizon of understanding shifts to a new horizon by an encounter with something new – this process named a 'fusion of horizons' is when the old and new horizons fuse and bring a renewed living value to our understanding.

3 'Being' and 'being' are used in this book to signal a distinction between the 'being' of entities, such as a chair, and 'Being' as existential. Heidegger (1927/1962) calls this the ontological difference, the crucial distinction between Being and beings. Unfortunately, the capitalisation of 'Being' can confuse. 'Being' is not itself a higher order

being waiting to be discovered but merely a way of signalling an essential distinction. The question of the meaning of Being is about what it is that makes beings (entities) intelligible as beings. Being is not itself simply another entity amongst other entities. That is Being is always the Being of some entity or being.

4 Dialectical in this context means the ability to view issues from multiple perspectives and arrive at the most plausible and reasonable understanding of seemingly contradictory and discordant information.

5 Technolust: a strong desire for and fascination with modern technology.

6 Self-actualisation according to Maslow is the linear progression towards a state of being that involves creative self-development in terms of one's potential towards a goal and a sense of meaning in life.

7 Peak experience is a state of heightened awareness. It can be compared to spiritual experiences but not necessarily. A peak experience can mean feeling high or humbled. The core experience is one of unity. For a full description, see Maslow (1964), pp. 59–68.

8 Details of the ethical process and approvals can be found on the open source copy of the PhD that includes the original ethics approval letter. Link: http://openrepository. aut.ac.nz/bitstream/handle/10292/7071/CrowtherS.pdf?sequence=3&isAllowed=y.

References

APPPH. (2013). *Birth Psychology*. Available at: http://birthpsychology.com/.

Barrett, A. (2017). Spiritual obstetrics. In: S. Crowther and J. Hall, eds, *Spirituality Childbirth: Meaning and Care at the Start of Life*. London: Routledge, pp. 133–141.

Bergum, V. and Van Der Zalm, J. (2007). *Motherlife: Studies of Mothering Experience*. Alberta, Canada: Pedagon Publishing.

Britton, J.R. (2012). The assessment of satisfaction with care in the perinatal period. *Journal of Psychosomatic Obstetrics & Gynaecology*, 33, pp. 37–44.

Caelli, K. (2001). Engaging with phenomenology: Is it more of a challenge than it needs to be? *Qualitative Health Research*, 11, pp. 273–281.

Campanelli, P. and Campanelli, D. (1998). *Pagan Rites of Passage*. St Paul, MN: Llewellyn Publications.

Cheyney, M. (2011). Re-inscribing the birthing body: Homebirth as ritual performance. *Medical Anthropology Quarterly*, 25, pp. 519–542.

Church, S. (2016). *New Thinking on Improving Maternity Care: International Perspectives*. London: Pinter & Martin Limited.

Crowther, S., Stephen, A. and Hall, J. 2019. Association of psychosocial–spiritual experiences around childbirth and subsequent perinatal mental health outcomes: an integrated review. *Journal of reproductive and infant psychology*, 1–26.

Crowther, S. (2016). Crafting stories in hermeneutic phenomenology research: A methodological device. *Qualitative Health Research*, 27(6), pp. 826–835.

Crowther, S. (2019). Birth and spirituality. In: Z. Laszlo and B. Flanagan, eds, *The Routledge International Handbook of Spirituality and Society*. London: Routledge, pp. 113–119.

Crowther, S. and Hall, J. (2017). *Spirituality and Childbirth: Meaning and Care at the Start of Life*. London and New York: Taylor & Francis.

Crowther, S., Smythe, E., and Spence, D. (2014). The joy at birth: An interpretive hermeneutic literature review. *Midwifery*, 30, pp. 157–165.

Dinkins, C. (2005). Shared inquiry: Socratic-hermeneutic interpre-viewing. In: P. Ironside, ed., *Beyond Method*. London: The University of Wisconsin, pp. 111–147.

Dixon, L., Skinner, J. and Foureur, M. (2013). The emotional journey of labour – Women's perspectives of the experience of labour moving towards birth. *Midwifery*, 30(3), pp. 371–377.

Doherty, M.E. (2010). Voices of midwives: A tapestry of challenges and blessings. *MCN The American Journal of Maternal/Child Nursing*, 35, pp. 96–101.

Downe, S., Finlayson, K., Oladapo, O., Bonet, M., Metin Gülmezoglu, A., and Norhayati, M.M. (2018). What matters to women during childbirth: A systematic qualitative review. *PloS One*, 13, p. e0194906.

Edwards, N. (2013). *Birthing Autonomy: Women's Experiences of Planning Home Births*. London and New York: Routledge.

Edwards, N., Mander, R., and Murphy-Lawless, J. (2018). *Untangling the Maternity Crisis*. London and New York: Taylor & Francis.

Fenwick, J., Staff, L., and Gamble, J. (2010). Why do women request caesarean section in a normal, healthy first pregnancy? *Midwifery*, 26, pp. 394–400.

Forbes-Rogers, T. (1966). *The Midwife and the Witch*. New Haven: Yale University Press.

Gadamer, H.G. (1960/1975). *Truth and Method*. New York: Seabury.

Gadamer, H.G. (2008/1967). *Philosophical Hermeneutics*. London: University of California Press.

Gaskin, I.M. (1977). *Spiritual Midwifery*. Summertown, TN: The Book Publishing Company.

Grigg, C.P., Tracy, S.K., Schmied, V., Daellenbach, R., and Kensington, M. (2015). Women's birthplace decision-making, the role of confidence: Part of the Evaluating Maternity Units study, New Zealand. *Midwifery*, 31, pp. 597–605.

Harrison, J.A. (2010). *Joy as Attunement and End in the Philosophies of Martin Heidegger and Henri Bergson*. Chicago, IL: The Faculty of the Graduate School, Loyola University of Chicago.

Heidegger, M. (1927/1962). *Being and Time*. New York: Harper.

Heidegger, M. (1971/2001). *Poetry, Language, Thought*. New York: HarperCollins.

Hennessey, A.M. and Davis-Floyd, R.E. (2018). *Imagery, Ritual, and Birth: Ontology between the Sacred and the Secular*. Lanham, MD: Lexington Books.

Holten, L. and de Miranda, E. (2016). Women' s motivations for having unassisted childbirth or high-risk homebirth: An exploration of the literature on 'birthing outside the system'. *Midwifery*, 38, pp. 55–62.

Joe. (2011). *The True Meaning of Bundle of Joy. New Dad Life: On My Way to Becoming a Father*. Available at: http://newdadlife.wordpress.com/2011/02/01/the-true-meaning-of-bundle-of-joy/.

Kennell, J.H. and Klaus, M.H. (1998). Bonding: Recent observations that alter perinatal care. *Pediatrics in Review/American Academy of Pediatrics*, 19, pp. 4–12.

Koch, T. (1996). Implementation of a hermeneutic inquiry in nursing: philosophy, rigour and representation. *Journal of Advanced Nursing*, 24, pp. 174–184.

Lahood, G. (2007). Rumour of angels and heavenly midwives: Anthropology of transpersonal events and childbirth. *Women and Birth*, 20, pp. 3–10.

Lokugamage, A. (2011). *The Heart in the Womb*. London: Docamali Limited.

Martin, C.H. and Fleming, V. (2011). The birth satisfaction scale. *International Journal of Health Care Quality Assurance*, 24, pp. 124–135.

Maslow, A. (1964). *Religions, Values and Peak Experiences*. Columbus: Ohio State University Press.

McAra-Couper, J., Jones, M., and Smythe, L. (2012). Caesarean-section, my body, my choice: The construction of 'informed choice' in relation to intervention in childbirth. *Feminism & Psychology*, 22, pp. 81–97.

Merleau-Ponty, M. (1962/2002). *The Phenomenology of Perception*. London: Routledge Classics.

Miles, M., Chapman, Y., Francis, K., *et al.* (2013). Exploring Heideggerian hermeneutic phenomenology: A perfect fit for midwifery research. *Women and Birth*, 26(4), pp. 273–276.

Paley, J. (2016). *Phenomenology as Qualitative Research: A Critical Analysis of Meaning Attribution*. London: Routledge.

Parratt, J. (2010). *Feeling like a Genius: Enhancing Women's Changing Embodied Self During First Childbearing*. Newcastle, NSW: Faculty of Health, School of Nursing and Midwifery, University of Newcastle.

Parse, R.R. (1997). Joy–sorrow: A study using the Parse research method. *Nursing Science Quarterly*, 10, pp. 80–87.

Pilkington, F.B. (2006). On Joy–sorrow: A paradoxical pattern of human becoming. *Nursing Science Quarterly*, 19, pp. 290–291.

Plested, M. and Kirkham, M. (2016). Risk and fear in the lived experience of birth without a midwife. *Midwifery*, 38, pp. 29–34.

Razak, A. (1990). Toward a womanist analysis of birth. In: I. Diamond and G.F. Orenstein, eds, *Reweaving the World: The Emergence of Ecofeminism*. San Francisco: Sierra Club Books, pp. 165–172.

Sawyer, A., Ayers, S., Abbott, J., Gyte, G., Rabe, H., and Duley, L. (2013). Measures of satisfaction with care during labour and birth: A comparative review. *BMC Pregnancy and Childbirth*, 13, pp. 108–108.

Schulkin, J., Morgan, M.A., and Rosen, J.B. (2005). A neuroendocrine mechanism for sustaining fear. *Trends in Neurosciences*, 28, pp. 629–635.

Smythe, E. (2005). The thinking of research: Philosophical conversations in healthcare research and scholarship. In: P. Ironside, ed., *Beyond Method*. Wisconsin: University of Wisconsin Press, pp. 223–258.

Smythe, E. (2010). Safety is an interpretive act: A hermeneutic analysis of care in childbirth. *International Journal of Nursing Studies*, 47, pp. 1474–1482.

Smythe, E. and Spence, D. (2012). Re-viewing literature in hermeneutic research. *International Journal of Qualitative Methods*, 11, pp. 12–25.

Tannen, D. (1998). *The Argument Culture: Moving from Debate to Dialogue*. New York: Random House.

Thomson, G. (2010). Psychology and labour experience: Birth as a peak experience. In: D. Walsh and S. Downe, eds, *Essential Midwifery Practice: Intrapartum Care*. Oxford: Wiley-Blackwell, pp. 191–212.

Thomson, G., Dykes, F., and Downe, S. (2011). *Qualitative Research in Midwifery and Childbirth: Phenomenological Approaches*. London: Routledge.

van Manen, M. (2014). *Phenomenology of Practice: Meaning-Giving Methods in Phenomenological Research and Writing*. Walnut Creek, CA: Left Coast Press.

Walsh, D. (2006). Subverting assembly-line birth: Childbirth in a free-standing birth centre. *Social Science and Medicine*, 62, pp. 1330–1340.

WHO. (2018). *WHO Recommendations: Intrapartum Care for a Positive Childbirth Experience*. Geneva: World Health Organization.

Winnicott, D.W. (1960). The theory of the parent–infant relationship. *International Journal of Psychoanalysis*, 41, pp. 585–595.

Wojtkowiak, J. and Crowther, S. (2018). An existential and spiritual discussion about childbirth: Contrasting spirituality at the beginning and end of life. *Spirituality in Clinical Practice*, 5, pp. 261–272.

2 Philosophical underpinnings

This chapter explores the main philosophical underpinnings that guided my thinking, ongoing analysis, and writing. Foregrounding philosophical underpinnings enables the reader to attune to hermeneutic phenomenological writings. The study used an interpretive hermeneutic phenomenological methodology informed principally from the works of Heidegger [1889–1976] and Gadamer [1900–2002]. The philosophical tenets of a hermeneutic phenomenology are inextricably linked to the study as a whole and thus embedded within the research project process itself. I do not claim to be a graduate of continental philosophy but use hermeneutic phenomenology as research method, maintaining that a grasp and appreciation of seminal writings in this philosophical tradition are necessary (Crowther, 2016). I contend that the integrity of a hermeneutic phenomenological study is held together by the connection to the underpinning philosophy. Therefore, this chapter is positioned early in the book because the philosophical tone of the chapters to follow is central to how the book is focused.

This study is ontologically focused. This means it is concerned with the study of existential 'Being' as distinguished from a study of entities or material objects. Put another way this study is not concerned with the material aspects of birth such as childbirth interventions, organisations of care, nor psychological or physical measurable outcomes (ontic as opposed to ontological, see Figure 2.1).

The challenge in describing this philosophical approach is that there is no one place to jump into the process of understanding. From my own experience it became quickly evident that hermeneutic phenomenology resonated with my own life view and experiences and how I orientated by questioning about childbirth. I realise that I found it incongruent with my own understanding and appreciation of childbirth to isolate aspects out of the whole as this fragmentation did not 'feel' right, neither did it focus on the human experiences that interested me. I found that how I questioned what is going on at birth was integral to who I am in the world (Gadamer, 2008/1967). I understood from my early tentative readings that this was 'my tradition' as this was already the way I engaged with the world around me including my professional interests in childbirth.

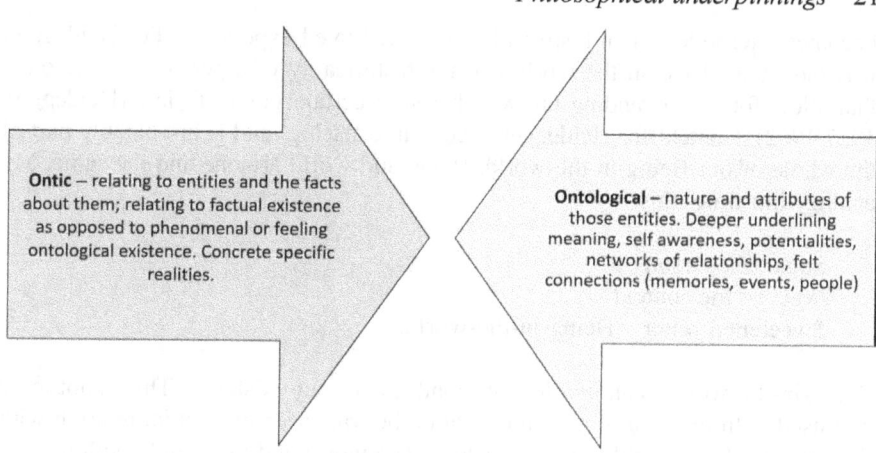

Figure 2.1 Ontic and ontological distinctions.

Tradition

Before I delve into exploring the philosophical notions underpinning this book some historical context to this approach to human inquiry is required. The history of the phenomenological movement has been associated with several eminent European philosophers that stretch back in time to Hegel [1770–1831] and Brentano [1838–1917]. However, it was Brentano's student Edmund Husserl [1859–1938] who is regarded as the father of phenomenology. Husserl confronted the scientific community for not acknowledging the human experience. He claimed that by ignoring this vital aspect of living subjects, scientific endeavours produced artificial de-contextualised findings because important variables were missed. Husserl's main focus was exploring how phenomena were revealed in consciousness. He was the first philosopher to openly challenge Cartesian mind body dualism (Husserl, 2001).

One of Husserl's pivotal ideas is that of intentionality in which the mind is directed towards objects. Another of his notions is bracketing or phenomenological reduction in which one puts aside the preconceptions and pre-understandings of the researcher. According to Husserl it was possible to remove outside distractions and personal biases from a study and its findings. Heidegger, Husserl's student, however, did not agree and broke from these central Husserlian notions. This is where the distinctiveness begins to show itself and is what drew me into Heideggerian thinking because the futility of attempting to somehow extract myself from the world I inhabited resonated with me.

Heidegger turned his focus from epistemological questions of knowing to ontology and the study of being itself in lived-experience, seeking meaning and sense of understanding. He used the term Dasein – 'Being-there' – to describe being open and intrinsically related to the world (Sheenan, 2000). This is the sense of 'I' that knows that it exists and is of issue to itself. Unlike Husserl, Heidegger understood consciousness and the world as inseparable entities. Consciousness thus becomes interpreted as an historical constructed lived-experience. For Heidegger, it is the situatedness in the world and the historicality of a person's background that allow for understanding the world from a certain point of view (Heidegger, 1927/1962). Context for Heidegger is central to 'Being' and is inseparably part of the whole of our Being-in-the-world. Being and world are one and the same. My analogy illustrates this:

Sugar = a person
Water = the context
Sweetened water = Being-in-the-world.

Being-in-the-world is an involuntary condition of our existence. This is not to be confused with the idea of a spatial relation but rather an existential relation with the entities of the world (Dreyfus, 1991). The world and the people within it are 'the world'. Being-in-the-world of birth is thus always a unitary phenomenon. The use of hyphens in Heideggerian notions emphasises this unitary nature of phenomena.

Heidegger identified two modes of Being-in-the-world as 'present-at-hand' and 'ready-to-hand' (Heidegger, 1927/1962). Present-at-hand modes of being are not how things in the world are normally encountered in everyday life. In this mode of Being things become separated from the relational whole of Being-in-the-world. The sugar is separated from the water following the previous analogy. Ready-to-hand is a more primordial ontological mode of being. It is the background familiarity that rarely comes to awareness. Yet, when ready-to-hand things in the world break down they become unready-to-hand, such as the door that gets stuck or the computer that suddenly powers down! The broken-down things come to awareness as present-to-hand; the broken lock on the door or the computer that just crashed need fixing. The door as a passage to another room and the computer that is a tool to write this book become stripped of their pre-reflective ready-to-hand mode of being. To illustrate further, the keys on my computer came into focus for the first time today as I tapped frantically to get the computer to reboot when it unexpectedly crashed. Until then it was part of a backgrounded whole relational world of authoring this book.

Meaning is always in the context of the interrelated notion of Being-in-the-world and is the standpoint for all understanding. Activities and events unfolding in the world reveal meaningful and significant encounters. However, meaning can be submerged in the background of Being-in-the-world as things become unnoticed and taken-for-granted. Therefore, to bracket or in some way to attempt to separate my understandings from their context and my own pre-understandings is impossible. As Koch (1996) explains, and the above sugar water analogy illustrates, there is an indissoluble unity between the world and people. My life, professionally and personally, is always already with me in the world. The traditions of phenomenology and hermeneutics are themselves in and of the world. Furthermore, they are not stationary; they come from a rich and textual thinking history that continues to evolve. Gadamer (1960/1975) maintained that such methodology is not fixed but continually open to new insights and possibilities. I remember clearly in a doctoral supervisory session being advised not to take fixed positions nor accept any philosophical notions as finalised but to work with them and allow other possibilities to be uncovered.

We are seemingly programmed to impose patterns where, perhaps, there are none. One may start looking for things that support that pattern and interpret findings accordingly; rather like scientific theories that fit the facts, except for the anomalies! The need to explain everything by assigning a final or root cause to all phenomenon can lead to premature declaration of absolute immutable truths; a thesis hard to defend in health and social sciences. Seeking universal laws and pursuit of teleological explanations (i.e. explanations based on the consideration of the 'ends' or 'goals' of things) can be limiting. As such the methodology of this inquiry evolved as has my own reflexive thinking and interpretations matured.

What is phenomenology?

Heideggerian phenomenology is fundamentally about Being and not about theories, ideas, and problem solving. Phenomenology as a research method is an invitation to observe and collect data pertaining to people's experience of lifeworld phenomena. It is a method for uncovering what lies hidden. Phenomenology is descriptive, focusing on the structures of experience seeking to surface meanings of lived-experiences (van Manen, 1997). Phenomenology in this inquiry focused on the lived-experience of the *phenomenon* 'joy at birth'.

What is a phenomenon?

Phenomenon, according to Heidegger, is that which is essentially withdrawn, hidden, forgotten, covered up, and even disguised (Heidegger, 1927/1962). In other words, phenomena are always covered over and can only ever be partially uncovered. Phenomena are taken-for-granted in the everyday familiar backgrounds that are pre-reflective and often unnoticed, like the crashed computer and the stuck door. To examine and bring to awareness this background in its wholeness is not possible and relates to the Heideggerian notion of truth that is always an on-the-way un-concealing.

The Greek word alétheia ($\dot{\alpha}\lambda\dot{\eta}\theta\varepsilon\iota\alpha$) used by Heidegger to mean truth includes the notion of un-concealment. Truth is not mere agreement or/and correctness but, in Heideggerian terms, a un-concealment of that which was hidden, covered up, forgotten (Heidegger, 1927/1962). Human beings (Daseins) are both in truth and untruth in a dialectical play. Truth is thus an un-concealing of phenomenon not some absolute definitive response to an inquiry. Heidegger's allegory shows Dasein's constant dialectical movement:

> The goddess of truth who guides Parmenides, puts two pathways before him, one of hiding; but this signifies nothing else than that Dasein [human being] is already both in truth and in untruth.

(1927/1962: 265)

Phenomena reveal themselves as appearance which is as close to the thing in itself as we will ever get. For example, smiling with joy at birth is a hint of background joy yet the smiling is not the joy itself. Joy itself is not revealed entirely and remains both revealed and covered up. Phenomena can also announce themselves, for example, "I feel so overcome with joy!" or as this author declares, "Birth is a fantastic connecting celebration of life … it's something I look forward to and look back on with great joy. I consider myself blessed to be allowed to participate in something so amazing and miraculous" (Schneider, 2012: 220). Phenomena can show themselves as semblance when what seems to be joy is something else. For example, a woman after birth cries at the birth of her son not with joy but with tears of sadness that her recently deceased mother would never meet her grandson. Heidegger explains:

> The uncovering of anything new is never done on the basis of having something completely hidden but takes its departure rather from uncoveredness in the mode of semblance. Entities look as if … that is, they have, in a certain way, been uncovered already, and yet they are still disguised.
>
> (1927/1962: 265)

Semblance cannot be the complete phenomenon itself because tears are not the essence of joy. The tears may point to something still concealed. Thus, the Being of phenomenon is always there but hidden, remaining unintelligible in such a state. This gestures to what Heidegger names circumspection.

Circumspection describes taken-for-granted everyday doing and experiencing in the world of birth. It is the coping and dealing with what is invisible, withdrawn, and transparent in that world. Much of the literature that I read prior and during the inquiry was concerned with the material, measurable or ontical. For example, babies are born in all locations and safety and judicious use of birthing technology is important but the lived-experience of Being-there at birth (wherever that physically happens) often remains invisible, withdrawn, and silenced. I was therefore constantly seeking the phenomenon 'joy at birth' that was disguised and hidden in the unnoticed circumspective background at birth.

The good news for a phenomenologist is that a phenomenon can be disclosed or unconcealed by reflection upon it making it explicit and seen, even though something of that phenomenon will always remain concealed. What is possible in our phenomenological inquiry is to attempt a plausible thematising of phenomena which brings them into language. This inquiry focused on pointing out the background or familiarity of birth and revealing understanding of the phenomenon 'joy at birth' that seemed hidden yet also near.

What is hermeneutics?

Hermeneutics is the study of meanings, relationships, and thinking upon relationships in context; it is not a study of objects separate from the whole (Gadamer, 1960/1975). Hermeneutics seeks to explicate and reveal inner meaning of human lived-experiences and is the art and skill of interpreting and understanding of such meanings. Gadamer emphasised a more practical application of hermeneutic phenomenology and informed much of the process of this study. In Truth and Method, his major work, Gadamer (1960/1975) articulated a philosophical approach that highlighted the conditions through which understanding itself takes place. 'Hermeneutics' and 'phenomenology' of Heidegger and Gadamer underpin an evolving methodology that can be utilised 'as research method' in the pursuit of human understanding.

What is hermeneutic phenomenological as research method?

Hermeneutic phenomenology as research method in health and social sciences is used when the research question seeks meanings of a phenomenon that intends to disclose understanding of a human experience (Crist and Tanner, 2003). However, we need to be prudent in labelling this journey as a method of fixed rules and processes. As Smythe (2019) suggests it is not a method that can be fully explicated, as some may try, but requires a trust in the process and a willingness to be inspired by the seminal writers of hermeneutics and phenomenology. As such this 'method' does not seek to construct labels of phenomena contributing to discourse, but rather reveal the meanings of Being-there or Dasein as an ontological enquiry. From within life, life is questioned, and it is hermeneutic phenomenology as an unbounded research method that lets things show themselves relationally. This corresponded with the guiding question of this study.

What is the experience of joy at the birth of a baby and how is this joy significant and meaningful?

Inherent in questions of lived-experience is a desire to reveal meaning and to understand the human experience, in this case birth from the perspective of those present in that moment. The methodology and goals of my study flowed directly from my initial research question. Although the initial question led to the philosophy, the philosophical lens consequently both influenced and guided the questions asked of the data and helped reveal the interpretations, relationships, and understandings. The philosophical underpinnings of hermeneutic phenomenology provided an opening into the lived-experience of joy at birth. Through the application of a hermeneutic interpretive phenomenological lens, I became sensitised to the different human ways of Being-in-the-world of birth.

The purpose of using hermeneutic phenomenology as research method was not to generate theories, solve problems, present generalizations, or develop a way of predicting the phenomenon joy at birth. The purpose was to describe the experience of attunement at birth and uncover meanings of such lived-experience whether it was joy or another attunement. Both experience and meaning were sought. The phenomenological approach provided an avenue to delve deeper into the human lived-experience of joy at birth whilst the meanings that may have been forgotten within such experiences were revealed through sustained exploration and questioning of this phenomenon hermeneutically.

There is a plethora of Heideggerian and Gadamerian notions. In this work particular emphasis is placed on Heidegger's understanding of Being as a foundation to interpretation and his notion of attunement (mood) as shared experience. In addition, Gadamer's hermeneutics draws attention to how text and understandings interact with the investigator's interpretations through the 'fusion of horizons' (Gadamer, 1960/1975). Both philosophers emphasised the reciprocity and contextual unity of phenomena that is central to this inquiry. Some specific philosophical notions are explored in order to situate the following chapters.

Dasein and mortals

The words Dasein and mortals are used interchangeably to describe human beings who are always engaged in the world in some way. The German word Dasein means, simply translated, 'Being-there' or an openly engaged human-being. Dasein, according to Heidegger (1927/1962), is an aspect of Beingness that is able to inquire and wonder about its own existence or its Being-there of existence. It is that sense of I that is at issue with itself. The reciprocal movement between things in the world and mortals (us) contributes to meaning in a relational interconnected totality. Dasein (human being), by its nature, lives life relationally with-others. Dasein is thus interpreting and existing hermeneutically due to its always already being-in-the-world. It is evident when considering this understanding that any attempt of 'bracketing' or setting aside who we are is futile.

Dasein (or human being) can be understood as being constituted by several existentials[1] that include temporality (felt-time), spatiality (felt-space), embodiment (felt-body), and relationality (felt-other). Dasein refers to an openness to possibility so it was crucial to always remain open to the possibility that Dasein (being human) at birth could be different and more than that found in the philosophical literature. For example, as I said above, other existential or philosophical notions were always possible, and an openness and constant return to the phenomenon itself is required.

Thrownness

Dasein is also always thrown somehow. We are thrown in our lives; this is an inescapable attribute of our Being-there (Dasein) (Heidegger, 1927/1962). For example, we are thrown into our family, our culture, and history at birth. I am thrown into moments of birth as a midwife as I am thrown into a world of maternity services. This thrownness is not referring to brute fact or the factuality of a concrete historical situation but rather that something already informs our existence and is often unnoticed and unattended. We also do not know how we are thrown into situations. For example, we do not fully know **how** we are thrown into a moment(s) at birth. I am currently thrown into writing this book, although I may have some sway over certain aspects of that writing experience. I am also thrown into a world of publisher's deadlines, regulations, editing rules, and relationships with editors. At the time of writing I am also thrown into the political turmoil of a Europe dealing with Brexit whilst engaging with the logistics of relinquishing my professorial chair in Aberdeen, Scotland and re-migrating

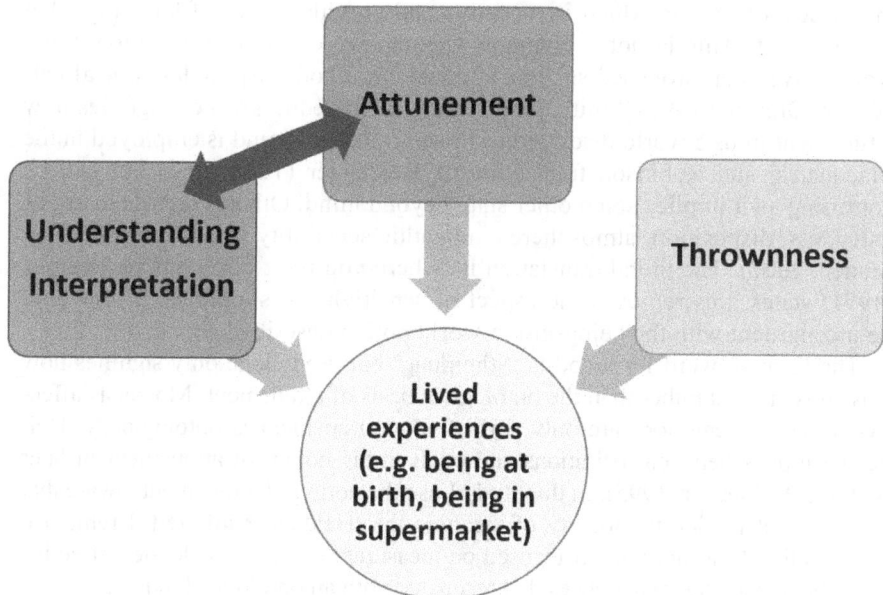

Figure 2.2 Attunement and throwness.

home to New Zealand. Equally, as a professor of midwifery, I am caught up in the values and practices of the midwifery profession and the complexities of being in a senior academic role. Some throwness can be dramatic and easily demarcated from everyday life, like being thrown into a birthing environment, some of our throwness is part of our everyday activities such as being 'thrown' into the busyness of a supermarket to buy dinner on the way home from work. What is key to understand here is how we are always thrown and how that throwness is non-volitional. Making our throwness intelligible is the purpose of Dasein's attunement (see Figure 2.2).

Attunement and mood

As Figure 2.2 illustrates our throwness is disclosed through Dasein's attunements or how it attunes to certain moods. It is the attunement of that world (e.g. the world of being a professor, being in the supermarket, being at birth) which discloses how we make sense of it. I have used Heidegger's notion of attunement to access the phenomenon of something special at birth, in this case a 'joy' that is complex to articulate. In-depth interpretations of this central notion are thus integral to the chapters that will follow. It was attunement at birth that claimed my attention at the start of this inquiry. Grappling with a hunch that something shared and significant was 'going on' at births, I was inspired by Heidegger's notion of attunement and could see that it provided a gateway into what I understood as shared experience at birth.

There are however several issues when using this notion, not least the translation issues. Heidegger uses the German word 'Befindlichkeit' to describe that aspect of Dasein which is receptive and provides ways of knowing what matters to it. This is not a common German word and in translation many words have been proposed such as attunement, mood, disposedness or affectedness (Dreyfus, 1991). Smith (1981) suggests findedness which signifies how attunement finds a world disclosed to Dasein. State-of-mind is employed in the Macquarrie and Robinson translation of Heidegger (1927/1962) but can be confusing as it implies some other state beyond mind. Other words such as situatedness, disposition, atmosphere, and pathic sensibility have been used (van Manen, 2007). The literal translation is 'where-you're-at-ness' but, as Dreyfus (1991) states, this removes the aspect of sensitivity to situations. This would be incongruent with the being-in-the-world notion described above.

The German word for mood is 'Stimmung' but used alone only signifies how Dasein is attuned rather than the ontological basis of attunement. Moods as affective states and emotions are only part of what attunement is ontologically. Heidegger moves between definitions and evolved his notion of attunement in later writings (Heidegger, 1995). In this study I use the notion of attunement, aware that this may not imbibe the totality of meaning that Heidegger inferred. I remained cautious that I did not remain focused on measurable and easily defined affective states but existential experiences that resonated with an ontological inquiry.

Attunement is an ontologically descriptive notion that is made concrete in affective states, such as moods and emotions that can be shown to have causes, such as fear of childbirth and are material, measurable, and often visible (e.g. ontic moods). Conversely, examining an ontological background of attunements is to foreground ontic (material) moods and appreciate attunement as the backgrounded basis upon which ontic moods manifest. In other words, attunement is the background workings of Dasein. Daseins are always attuned somehow, making the foregrounded ontic affective states including moods and emotions possible. In other words, attunements are not merely passing personal feelings or emotions but are intrinsically a part of the shared experience of Being-in-the-world, namely, Dasein and human being.

Attunement can refer to the individual attuned state as well as the cultural sensibility or mood of the times and thus provides a context that governs the possibility of other moods (Dreyfus, 1991). Attunements are thus a shared communication and not necessarily private. They can be social and public and represent ways of Being-with-one-another. They provide a sense of collective and personal experience of how a situation is unfolding and how we are faring; a public shared communication that reveals the situated experiences of our thrownness, such as being at birth. Yet there are instances in which an individual may not share the collective mood, failing to attune to the atmosphere of the moment. For example, the depressed person who arrives for an upbeat celebratory dinner with friends. Nonetheless, Heidegger contends:

> Dasein always has some mood. The pallid, evenly balanced lack of mood, which is often persistent, and which is not to be mistaken for a bad mood, is far from nothing at all.
>
> (Heidegger, 1927/1962: 173)

It is possible to turn towards or away from attunements but, in turning away, one is attuned to another as Dasein is always attuned somehow. We are thus always tuned into the things that matter to us as the *tuning in* is our mood (Blattner, 2006; Smith, 1981). Attuning to something that matters to us in our thrownness thus awakens attunement to allow lived-experiences, such as joy at birth, to become intelligible to us. However, according to Heidegger it is not possible to verify an attunement we can only draw attention to it and awaken it:

> ... we shall not speak at all of ascertaining a fundamental attunement in our philosophizing, but of awakening it. Awakening means making something wakeful, letting whatever is sleeping become wakeful.
>
> (Heidegger, 1995: 60)

This is an important point when we come to think about how some births that appear to lack joy for a variety of reasons (Crowther *et al.*, 2014). Exploring attunements and naming them can be challenging because they are only dis-closed in a pre-reflective way (Dreyfus, 1991), yet they set the tone on how we interpret events in which we are thrown into. So how can we study these elusive attunements? Heidegger asserts that attunements are only uncovered in times of breakdown. This can be used to our advantage in phenomenological work because when there is breakdown, in this case in birth experiences, attunements can be awoken so that they become visible.

Overall, attunements open mortals (human beings) to forward possibilities and help us interpret and understand the world we are thrown into, often unknowingly (Heidegger, 1927/1962). Moreover, existential attunements open the shared world up to possibilities. For example, the shared jollity of the cele-bratory dinner party could open possibilities towards making new connections with others that would not normally be in the circle of contacts of everyday life; the depressed sad mood could be replaced with joy. Attunements thus provide opportunities that open to possibilities not yet known.

Heidegger describes fundamental-grounding attunements or Grundstim-mung. Grounding attunements orientate us to the world, investing that world with significance that shapes perspectives of that world. These are basic attunements that Heidegger calls irruptions that are all pervasive, intense, and overwhelming. Such attunements do not just colour our world but take us over and alter its structure, carry us away beyond ourselves, and change the way we view the world in profound ways. Battaly (2011) refers to this as a totalising attunement that organises our world into a whole that is meaningful. Heidegger says such attunements "can occur out of the blue, and precisely whenever we do not expect it at all" (Heidegger, 1995: 135). This last insight is key to understanding attunements as more than passing affective states but something foundational and basic in the experience of Being-there at birth.

Heidegger argues that some moods are basic passions and constitute Dasein. For example, Heidegger (1961/1981) speaks of love as a basic passion. Passion can be revealed through powerful emotions, such as love, joy, hatred, or anger. Speaking about the passion of love Heidegger says:

> Love is never blind: it is perspicacious. Only infatuation is blind, fickle, and susceptible – an affect, not a passion. To passion belongs a reaching out and opening up of oneself ... reaching out in passion does not simply lift us up and away beyond ourselves. It gathers our essential Being to its proper ground, it exposes our ground for the first time in a gathering, so that the passion is that through which we take hold of ourselves and achieve lucid mastery of the beings around us and within us.
>
> (1961/1981: 47–48)

Heidegger's analytic of attunement and passion are far reaching and open us to the possibility that within our experiences (such as being at birth) there is the possibility of an "ancient something which conceals itself" (Heidegger, 2002: 24). This gestures to an existential longing in Heidegger's work on Schelling where a sense of silenced inner longing for rootedness and belonging gets nearer to a self-concealed self (Heidegger, 1985). It also touches on Rudolf Otto's (1917/1923) notion of the numinous and Schelling's upsurgence of yearning in the ground of God (Heidegger, 1985). These philosophical writings reminded me of the vastness of how joy as a possible grounding attunement at birth is experienced and interpreted, arriving like a messenger to gift deeper understandings about life. What is evident is how mood or attunement of situations that we find ourselves thrown into, such as being at birth, calls us to respond.

Messengers, hints and gestures

Heidegger's (1982) later work used the terms messengers, hints, and gestures and these are central to this study. For Heidegger, gesture is a pointing out of something that may not be obvious but calls to us as hints. A gesture can point beyond human experience to something ineffable that shows itself from within experience as hints. A gesture announces that something is coming. For example, the gesture of birth perhaps hints at something special arriving. Hint, according to Heidegger, is also a call to questioning that unveils what confounds us as human beings. A hint never provides the final answer, it merely signals a possible way forward.

The hint that beckoned me to questioning at the start of this study was something ineffable that provoked a desire in me to know more about the nature of Being at birth and what meanings it held. This hint left a trace from wherever it came. Simply put, I was left with a hunch. Hints thus arrive in response to a desire to understand something in an open and receptive manner. They do not come from the receiver but the phenomenon itself which calls out. Hints beckon, invoke, and encourage thinking.

Individual stories will be presented in the following chapters and act as messengers of the phenomenon that hint at something. The messages from participant interviews, a hermeneutic literature review, listening to others at conferences, and within my own work and personal day to day life coalesced into greater understanding through myriad hints of what the messages sought to convey. I came to see that everything messages; both words and attunements were messengers. They all left me with a trace of themselves in their gifting. Ultimately, it was not the individual stories themselves but common meaning that surfaced that forever changed how the phenomenon was understood.

Mortals are always connected to the giver of the message as that is what makes it a gift. Both giver and receiver are left with a trace of each other. In the gift of the disclosure, a trace of the giver remains. Without that remaining trace it is never a gift, for it is not possible to fully appropriate anything. Mortals are, however, touched and affected by these gifts and are grateful. I was touched and grateful for the gifts given in the data collection of this study. Like a loved one who gives a gift as a gesture of affection that hints at their concern for you; there is a connection. As receiver of the gift I retained traces of the giver. Likewise, the giver of the gift retained a trace of the gift. As I responded to the messages, I was left with traces that connected me with something just beyond language that invoked more questions. This indefinable quality at birth is something that I was deeply concerned about. Similarly, I suspect as a reader of this book you are concerned either about birth or/and this methodology from your unique perspective. I assume you would not come to reading this page disengaged and disinterested in the content!

Structure of care

According to Heidegger we are always concerned with something. Thus, our basic structure of involvement in the world is 'care'; only in a dis-interested mode do we become disengaged, disinterested, or negligent observers. Care and concern, in this context, are expressed through action and not to be confused with an emotive state. Care as providing comfort and assistance is something that arises from the ontological notion of concern. Concern is a characteristic of existence which makes visible who we are as care. Being-in-the-world is to care, and care is synonymous with Dasein's Being and actions (Heidegger, 1927/1962). In care's positive mode, we always care about things somehow and in some way in the world. We are all mattering to each other in variable ways, in other words, I can be enthusiastic in my approach to caring or I can be dis-interested or negligent in my care.

Care, in this context, is not concerned worrying but care of something that matters (or not). Defining Dasein's Being as care and therefore Being-with-others relationally is the fundamental way of Dasein understanding. Caring is thus a derivative of our actions to actualise mutual plans in our worlds. I am reminded of my own primary characteristic of Being-in-the-world as midwife-researcher and my involvements with the concerns in that world with others and how they are expressed as care. The concern we have of Being-with-others and how we are comported in the world is akin to solicitude (Heidegger, 1927/1962). Solicitude is revealed further in the following chapters.

Understanding and interpretation

There is recognition and acceptance in hermeneutic interpretive phenomenology that those involved in research are inextricably situated in their worlds. According to Heidegger (1927/1962) any interpretations are influenced by our fore-structures of understanding, including our history and traditions, and cannot be removed from our unfolding understandings. In hermeneutics the subject and object are in continuous dialogue until there is a fusion and the boundaries between begin to dissolve. Gadamer (1960/1975) further asserts that every researcher has prejudices, a culture, and a fore-structure. The fore-structure of understanding is a template consisting of fore-having, fore-sight, and fore-conception. This tripartite structure is the basis of interpretation and understanding (Heidegger, 1927/1962).

Heidegger's three fore-structures of understanding constitute the basis of interpretations. Fore-having is the pre-understanding or judgements that I have in advance due to my historical and cultural background. It is the interpretation grounded in the context of my life that I had in advance of commencing this research. Fore-sight includes the seeing something *as* something, such as birth as special or sacred. The interpretive or hermeneutic 'as' recognises that a phenomenon is understood as something – in this case, birth specialness as potentially spiritual and sacred. I had suspected this meaning in advance of interpreting the data. Fore-conception is how I understand and how I was led to the questions asked and what I, in advance, conceptualised and expected to find. I held conceptions of the phenomenon that were grasped in advance.

Pre-understandings and reflexivity

In relation to this my own pre-understandings or prejudices required continual identification. Pre-understandings are inextricably part of this inquiry. This was vital to understanding the dialectical nature of the endeavour and to achieve clarity and integrity of the inquiry. Using a Heideggerian approach to phenomenology I was not required to bracket and put aside my own pre-understandings or theories as suggested by Husserl's (2001) transcendental phenomenology. On the contrary, the process included the significance of the existing lived world and its meanings that I find myself thrown into as human being – midwife, midwifery educator, and researcher.

As researcher I brought my thinking to a phenomenon that continually disclosed itself from the phenomenon itself to me. My thinking, and what was being disclosed, fused and evolved understanding. I was not separate from this Being-in-the world of birth and this contributed to the creative unfolding methodology. Phenomenology was the seeing and experiencing of the joy at birth and the hermeneutic understanding acknowledged that I was always already in the world of birth interpreting and bringing meaning. This is also influenced by what Heidegger termed the voice of the One or dictatorial They.

The One is the faceless tide of public opinion and values around birth that leads to conformity or non-conformity. The One is not construed as negative but an aspect of our Being-in-the-world with others. Heidegger (1927/1962) contends that surrendering ourselves to the voice of the One is problematic. To be aware and question the dictates of the One is a more authentic way of Being-in-the-world that reveals further possibilities. Although Heidegger recognises that both authentic and inauthentic ways of Being are part of Dasein, to be authentic is to be present and fully aware and engaged and not fallen into the dictates of the One. To be authentic, according to Heidegger, would enable genuine understanding of contextual complexity in which lived-experiences unfold.

Historical effective consciousness

Gadamer (1960/1975) asserts that our pre-understandings/prejudices are not only existential or ontological but also fully inserted within tradition. Midwifery and childbirth come with their historical consciousness, revealing an historical horizon of the birthing human experience as it is now:

> In fact, history does not belong to us; we belong to it. Long before we understand ourselves through the process of self-examination, we understand ourselves in a self-evident way in the family, society, and state in which we live.
>
> (Gadamer, 1960/1975: 278)

All my pre-understandings were thus historically limited and linked to my prejudices of the phenomenon influencing my interpretations and understandings. Prejudices are often paradoxical and oppositionally coexist as enabling or limiting, true or false:

> True prejudices facilitate further understanding while false prejudices hinder such development. Prejudices originate from past experiences and influence future possibility. They enable us to make sense of the situations in which we find ourselves, yet they also constrain understanding and limit the capacity to come to new and different ways of being. It is this contradiction that makes prejudice paradoxical ... accepting the notion of paradox is therefore a means of keeping tensions alive and possibilities open.
>
> (Spence, 1999: 163–164)

My pre-understandings were not merely abstract or ontological but part of the birthing and midwifery tradition made up of that history. This was part of my fore-structured understanding; my involvement in birth is always based on subjective prejudice. Enabling and recognising prejudices allowed for openness and receptivity; it kept the questioning dynamic so that possibilities could unfold. Limiting my prejudices would not honour difference and newness, potentially restricting the emergence of novel alternative understandings. This is not just a subjective meaning of the historical because my prejudices were not only embedded in the history of the tradition of birthing and midwifery but provoked by my ontological questioning.

This historical horizon was not just about the history handed down to me and others about childbirth but how I interpreted and responded to my day to day lived-experience. As historical effected mortals, past understandings meet us in the present and thus influence how experiences are interpreted. As Gadamer reminds us, "Our historical consciousness is always filled with a variety of voices in which the echo of the past is heard" (1960/1975: 285). I understood that I was in a world informed by the actions of those that had been before that shaped my contemporary personal beliefs and understandings in order that the phenomenon became intelligible to me. This was unavoidable as prejudices are required to open up to what is to be understood. Prejudices are therefore construed positively; they are pre-judgements of the phenomenon studied that are able to change. They are the starting point of investigation and provoke questioning from a certain point of view including interrogation of these personally held pre-judgements themselves.

It was imperative to keep questioning in order to enable open engagement with the phenomenon and not become rigid so that new understandings could surface. For example, midwifery has a history involving political and professional status struggles. It holds a perspective on birth as a social and normal life event that involves relationships and partnerships. This history and these beliefs are central to my midwife view to birth today. Yet there is also the history of the women's movement, evolution of obstetrics, and anthropological horizons – to name a few – that contribute to the way birth is enacted today. These horizons are explored further in the following chapter.

Historicity[2] is a closely bound up relationship one with the past and the present; one is bound to the other. The historical horizon of conscious Beings is in the world and can appear to be limiting. Yet, Gadamer (1960/1975) contends that understanding of contemporary experiences and their historicity results in a fusion that contributes to a more comprehensive understanding of the present. I acknowledged the messages of the past whilst remaining conscious not to be totally thrown into that historical perspective. This would have left me unreceptive to the messages and hints from the phenomenon of the experience as it is in front of me now.

Engagement with the historical horizons opened up ways to view that which was unfamiliar. I was able to move beyond and see things that did not sit well in my initial knowing of attunement at birth. Further understandings and deeper meanings hidden within – and part of traditions that inform twenty-first century birthing practices – were able to surface and join my thinking. My past met me continually in the present and was part of the understanding that made up the flow of spiralling interpretations. As researcher, educator, and practising midwife I therefore had a sense of what matters; a hunch and prior understanding. Gadamer calls this prior understanding our historical effective consciousness "... an element in the act of understanding itself ... (that) ... is already effective in finding the right questions to ask" (Gadamer, 1960/1975: 301). As natal beings we are all affected by birth and thus, distantly or intimately, always in and around birth somehow. The phenomenon of joy at birth messaged and hinted towards something. I was therefore affected and touched by the world I live in as a natal being and a midwife and compelled to question.

Gadamer suggests that disclosure of my own interpretations and pre-understandings helps to develop awareness of my prejudices. This is an iterative process that deepens the knowledge of what is known and what is being sought to know through a dialectical interplay between the parts and the whole. It was important to continually ensure that past, evolving, and present understandings were constantly questioned to further reveal the phenomenon.

With the above in mind, excavating and becoming clear about my pre-understandings or pre-judgements was crucial. Effective historical consciousness highlights how understanding emerges in the hermeneutic situation. Personal pre-understandings and evolving interpretations were collected in concurrent field notes, poems I wrote on the way, and a reflective diary, some of which appear in the chapters to follow. This is in order to show where I was coming from and how I was attuned and faring as I took this journey of inquiry.

Hermeneutic circle and fusion of horizons

The hermeneutic circle, or spiral as I would prefer to visualise the process, describes how one moves from the parts to the whole and the whole to the parts through a dialectical interplay (Gadamer, 1960/75). The notion of a hermeneutic circle was challenged by Heidegger in his later work. The circle became more expansive and relational with the mirroring of beings (ontic) and Being (ontological) in ways not articulated in the 1927 *Being and Time* (Heidegger, 1982). The reciprocity of relational interpretation was understood as a process that develops and grows; parts to whole, back and forth, constantly expanding. This more expansive and inclusive view shows how world – in this case world of birth – gifts messages, providing hints that take us to limits beyond that which is purely within our own capacity to understand and interpret. According to Gadamer the world and Dasein are in constant dialectic play. The world no longer depended on Dasein and things in the world were no longer purely purposeful objects for Dasein. There is reciprocity between the things of the world and Dasein which was not explicated in Heidegger's earlier work (Heidegger, 1971/2001, 1982).

The metaphor image of a circle is therefore limiting because the line of a circle always arrives back on itself. I found that the circle metaphor became a never-ending spiralling of expansion at the limits of endless possibility as the play unfolded. To spiral and expand in hermeneutic phenomenology work is never to arrive back at the start because we can no longer return to a 'start' that no longer exists. This was my experience. I was unable to return to my prior understandings; the inquiry process changed me on multiple levels. This inquiry was a dialectic of meaning, a scientific systematic path that built up deepening understandings according to my intention and ideological disposition as midwife researcher. For this I needed to remain both methodical and disciplined whilst dwelling in and working with the data as emerging horizons of understandings surfaced.

As you read this book your understandings will change, you will find yourself thrown into different possibilities as you ponder the content of the pages. The process of this way of working brings new insights and new experiences to the fore in an ever-evolving process as conflicts and readjustments to the new are brought into play. Laverty describes Gadamer's notion of horizon as:

> ... a range of vision that includes everything seen from a particular vantage point ... to have a horizon means being able to see beyond what is close at hand.
>
> (2003: 10)

This inquiry was a process of different horizons fusing that revealed a new wholeness that was more than the sum of its parts. The intention in the following pages is to present an experiential human phenomenon. The spiralling understanding of experience never ends yet articulating the meaning of a phenomenon within the context of research requires some form of ending. This was not an abrupt moment in time but a moment always on the way. This time was a time when contradictions in the data ceased and previously hidden meanings had been unconcealed, revealing a new horizon that was brought to language.

The end of this study was where I chose to step off. The interpretation of 'truth' was only revealed to the point I chose to finish. However, the thinking continued and weaved into these pages is my ongoing thinking and interpreting. Each time I come back to the original completed thesis, I come with wonder and see anew. The chapters that follow are an invitation to engage with the stories in a way that allows a bridging between your current limited horizons of understanding with those limited horizons of the stories and my interpretations of them for the sake of illuminating new appreciation of a phenomenon that is always at the same time concealed and unconcealed from us. Something in phenomenon remains always concealed even though parts become un-concealed. Phenomena are always in withdrawal, always partly hidden, never fully grasped. Bringing phenomena to language and interpreting exact meaning often remains elusive. A phenomenon plays between showing itself and hiding itself. It is never possible to get to the whole truth. The phenomenon of this study was no different, as you will discover in this book.

Conclusion

This chapter has introduced the philosophical underpinnings and explored the central notions that orientate us to the ontology of this inquiry. How we come to know anything and how understanding and interpretation arise together in human knowing has been highlighted. Reflexivity and the significance of foregrounding pre-understandings to a phenomenological inquiry have been explored by identifying the fore-structures of understanding that provide a background for subsequent interpretations. Bringing the phenomenon of this inquiry, 'joy at birth', to language demanded a methodology that would uncover the ontological experience and surface hidden meanings in a flexible yet systematically scientific way. Hermeneutic phenomenology as the philosophical basis for this inquiry provided the tools for engaging with the phenomenon and called me into sustained contemplative thinking that allowed something of significance to be un-concealed.

Returning to the notion of effective historical consciousness, the next chapter is a survey of material that contextualises this phenomenon historically and contemporaneously through the seen and unseen stories of joy at birth as it has evolved through the ages.

Notes

1 Existentials in this context relate to or affirm existential propositions and attributes of existence. Put another way they are those elements or constituent parts making up existence.
2 Historicity – A principle of understanding that explicates a reciprocal relation between understanding of history and tradition. The notion, from a hermeneutic perspective, addresses the gap between object and subject in human sciences' research and highlights our finite limited human understanding and foregrounds the ongoing reliance and contamination of knowledge from understandings of what has occurred previously (knowingly or unknowingly, consciously or unconsciously). This concerns our temporal existence and postulates an epistemological stance that suggests we are always our history, preconceptions, and judgements – we know what we know because we are historical beings.

References

Battaly, H. (2011). *Virtue and Vice, Moral and Epistemic.* London: John Wiley & Sons.
Blattner, W.D. (2006). *Heidegger's Being and Time: A Reader's Guide.* New York: Continuum International Publishing Group.
Crist, J.D. and Tanner, C.A. (2003). Interpretation/analysis methods in hermeneutic interpretive phenomenology. *Nursing Research,* 52, pp. 202–205.
Crowther, S. (2016). Crafting stories in hermeneutic phenomenology research: A methodological device. *Qualitative Health Research,* 27(6), pp. 826–835.
Crowther, S., Smythe, L., and Spence, D. (2014). Mood and birth experience. *Women and Birth: Journal of the Australian College of Midwives,* 27, pp. 21–25.
Dreyfus, H.L. (1991). *Being-in-the-World: A Commentary on Heidegger's Being and Time, Division I.* Cambridge, MA: MIT Press.
Gadamer, H.G. (1960/1975). *Truth and Method.* New York: Seabury.
Gadamer, H.G. (2008/1967). *Philosophical Hermeneutics.* London: University of California Press.
Heidegger, M. (1927/1962). *Being and Time.* New York: Harper.
Heidegger, M. (1961/1981). *Nietzsche: The Will to Power as Art.* London: Routledge & Kegan Paul.
Heidegger, M. (1971/2001). *Poetry, Language, Thought.* New York: HarperCollins.
Heidegger, M. (1982). A dialogue on language. In: *On the Way to Language.* San Francisco, CA: Harper and Row, pp. 1–54.
Heidegger, M. (1985). *Schelling's Treatise on the Essence of Human Freedom.* Columbus, OH: Ohio University Press.
Heidegger, M. (1995). *The Fundamental Concepts of Metaphysics: World, Finitude, Solitude.* Bloomington, IN: Indiana University Press.
Heidegger, M. (2002). *On Time and Being.* Chicago, IL: University of Chicago Press.
Husserl, E. (2001). *Logical Investigations.* London: Routledge.
Koch, T. (1996). Implementation of a hermeneutic inquiry in nursing: Philosophy, rigour and representation. *Journal of Advanced Nursing,* 24, pp. 174–184.

Laverty, S.M. (2003). Hermeneutic phenomenology and phenomenology: A comparison of historical and methodological considerations. *International Journal of Qualitative Methods*, 2, pp. 21–35.

Otto, R. (1917/1923). *The Idea of the Holy (Das Heilige)*. London: Oxford University Press.

Schneider, D.A. (2012). The miracle bearers: Narratives of birthing women and implications for spiritually informed social work practice. *Journal of Social Service Research*, 38, pp. 212–230.

Sheenan, T. (2000). Kehre and Ereignis: A prolegomenon to introduction to metaphysics. In: G. Fried and R. Polt, eds, *A Companion to Martin Heidegger's Introduction to Metaphysics*. New Haven, CT: Yale University Press, pp. 3–16.

Smith, Q. (1981). On Heidegger's theory of moods. *The Modern Schoolman*, 58, pp. 211–235.

Smythe, E. (2019). Commentary on: "A critical analysis of articles using a Gadamerian-based research method" (Fleming & Robb). *Nursing Inquiry*, 26, p. e12287.

Spence, D. (1999). *Prejudice, Paradox and Possibility: Nursing People from Cultures Other Than One's Own*. Auckland, NZ: Massey University.

van Manen, M. (1997). From meaning to method. *Qualitative Health Research*, 7, pp. 345–369.

van Manen, M. (2007). Phenomenology of practice. *Phenomenology & Practice*, 1, pp. 11–30.

3 Context and mood

All human experiences are culturally and historically determined, including birth. This chapter turns to the history, culture, and tradition through the use of myriad sources including literature, media, novels, and historical sources. It explores how our pre-understandings and collective effective historical consciousness constructs the world in which birth occurs. This chapter is not presented as a comprehensive historical rendition of all human birth across all cultures – that wouldn't be feasible or warranted – but instead offers glimpses of human birth from my own reading and thinking and focuses our gaze on the phenomenon that will be explored in the following chapters.

To explore any phenomenon at birth is at once to address all of birth, past and present, which at the same time is connected to future possibilities. Drawing out the changing moods concerning childbirth across time and cultures provides glimpses of significance and evidence of how those at birth are attuned. Heidegger tells us that entering the hermeneutic circle or spiral (see previous chapter) needs to be done in the right way. Setting the scene for this hermeneutic phenomenology study helps situate the inquiry as a whole and helps us enter the hermeneutic circle. Experiential stories taken from historical novels, theses, dissertations, anthropology, historical writings, movies, and television, as well as textbooks, open windows into different times and cultures.

Influences on birth-attunement

I argue, like others, that birth is not purely physiological but enmeshed in its own unique context (e.g. Delaporte and Martin, 2018; Hennessey and Davis-Floyd, 2018; Schneider, 2012; Callister and Khalaf, 2010; Cassidy, 2006; Clarke, 2012; Crouch and Manderson, 1993). Human civilisation has witnessed changes in the social and cultural context of birth. These changes involve continuing modification in symbolism (Hennessey and Davis-Floyd, 2018), behaviour, organisation of care, (Sandall *et al.*, 2016; Davis-Floyd, 2017; Homer *et al.*, 2019) and emergence of new value systems and how birth is narrated through a modern birth story (Kay *et al.*, 2017).

The influences on birth experience and attunement are dynamic and change reflecting social, religious, and emotional meanings. Birth is uniquely personal as well as societal. As Crouch and Manderson (1993), contend birth is a unique and significant occurrence for all those concerned and as a result the 'social significance, practices related to birth reflect salient cultural conditions and values and articulate these further within their own domain of meaning and reference' (56). As such, birth ideologies, medical or natural, comprise significant cultural and political discourses that reveal the effective dominant beliefs and ideas of a time and place. Over time values form images of the prevailing cultural and social interpretations become reflected in the stories told about birth (Kay *et al.*, 2017). An attunement (or mood) at birth is thus revealed within historical and cultural horizons contributing to how birth is understood.

The human birth story reveals an evolving multi-cultural and multi-historical spiralling that converges and diverges in meaning and practice. Some cultures appear to change faster than others. Some remain connected to ancient meanings depicted in birth ritual and practices. However, each aspect of the human birth story relates and builds upon the whole and uncovers something about how those present at birth attune. It is acknowledged that aspects of this history overlap and can be depicted in a different order. Furthermore, some themes flow through time without a defined beginning and end. Other more global influences from birth culture around the world are also acknowledged but are not the primary focus. This is only an overview demonstrating the enormous evolution of human thought that affects birth; a story that is still being played out daily at each birth globally.

The voice of the One shaping birth

There is a danger in a one-dimensional way of looking at birth; the western approach is only one of many views. Cross cultural and historical perspectives are essential in any attempt to reveal the attunement at birth. Ways of understanding the mystery of birth and its dangers are evident throughout human culture and history. A newborn baby can be a joy that is born through a precarious even dangerous process. This simple truth resonates through all cultures and through known history. Historically, birth has been cloaked in mystery associated with notions of sacredness, taboo, pollution, risk, and fear. Birth can be recognised as a liminal time of danger but also as one of communal joy. Many changes have occurred in the way birth is enacted through time and across cultures and passed to us in stories, pictures, and written material from a variety of sources.

Birth as social metaphor reflects how the dominant social context informs interpretations of birth. Each western society can be viewed as a unique blend of cultures and histories that merges with a global contemporary westernised birth culture that has changed over time. It could be construed that there is now a global birth culture with its own distinctive dictatorial voice of the One. I argue that the voice of the One (or dictorial They) resonates throughout the history of birth. Heidegger's notion of The One, introduced in the previous chapter, can be seen as shaping behaviour and practice that "... retains and enhances its stubborn dominion" (Heidegger, 1927/1962: 165). These are strong words and gesture to an inflexibility, restricting better care practices, research, and management strategies. This restrictiveness could give rise to individuals, and sometimes groups, working with birth outside of the voices of the They. Not to say these are in any way more authentic in their choices because the homebirth midwife and birthing women may be within the rhetorical discourses of '*normal birth only occurs at home without any medical interference*' – there is a significant lobby of birth activists (rightly or wrongly) who advocate this approach, equally obstetricians find themselves conforming to the One of medical discourse. In recent years, there has been a rise on reported births without professional health care assistance in the west (Holten and de Miranda, 2016), yet this phenomenon can also be attributed to the assailing mood of contemporary birthing which appears to embrace dichotomous thinking and practices. Phenomenology is not concerned with false dichotomous thinking but revealing meaning within experiences – whatever individual or group orientation.

Magical and sacred protection

Childbirth practices in primitive societies were probably informed by magical and supernatural beliefs as well as empirical experiences. Anthropological discoveries uncover birthing and dying as spiritual occasions from prehistoric times (Kitzinger, 2011). To this day myth and magic, ritual, sacred acts, and holy rites around birth continue to be found universally throughout human cultures (Hennessey and Davis-Floyd, 2018; Selin and Stone, 2009; Campanelli and Campanelli, 1998). The idea of birth being under the auspices of Earth Goddess and other female deities was strong (Crowley, 2001; Kitzinger, 2011; Hill, 2011). Women birthing may have called upon a feminine divine presence dwelling in the universe providing order and purpose. For example, the Gnostic gospels speak of God as Mother or Sophia (wisdom) who exists before all else. There is evidence that birth was interpreted as sacramental with spirits invited or/and sent away (Kitzinger, 2011; Selin and Stone, 2009).

Early and traditional creation stories tell of wonder and joyousness at the advent of new life across cultures (Selin and Stone, 2009), for example, Rimene and colleagues (1998) found complex belief systems around New Zealand Māori childbirth culture. Furthermore, support from others and belief in a holy other is found through early history and remains throughout many contemporary religious oral narratives (Callister and Khalaf, 2009). Birth practices that intended to spiritually protect birth potentially uncover something meaningful and perhaps sacred. Attuning to spiritual help and use of ritual aid continues in traditional birthing cultures today, for example, amongst Navajo people (Begay, 2009), Māori (Rimene *et al.*, 1998), Appalachian pregnant women (Jesse and Reed, 2004), Muslim women in an Arabian gulf state (Hanely and Brown, 2014), some Pagan followers (Campanelli and Campanelli, 1998), and Western women (Hennessey and Davis-Floyd, 2018).

Many of the birth practices and rituals in early birthing point to women as supporters with men only occasionally involved. The introduction of others at human birth is perhaps one of the earliest cultural birth practices as humans sought ways to ensure survival of their progeny. Bringing others to birth initiated practices and rituals that allowed cultural values, beliefs, sacred symbolism, and meanings to evolve.

Others at birth begins

The pain and anxiety associated with changing physiology brought others to birth. The altricial status[1] of human babies coupled with the evolutionary changes created what were previously only rare issues amongst mammals. There was discordance between the mammalian birth process and the speed of human evolution and changes in birth practices occurred (Trevathan, 1987). It has been suggested that bringing others to assist occurred as a response to the risks associated with bipedalism and increasing brain size. As such this need for assistance at human birth has become a necessity for survival (Davis-Floyd and Cheyney, 2009). Who these others were at birth has changed over time.

Birth as women's business

In ancient cultures the skill of midwives was essential to a community. Births would have been attended by known others, often women and sometimes shamans and/or traditionally skilled attendants (Begay, 2009; Clarke, 2012; Walsh, 2009). In rare cases, giving birth alone and away from the domestic situation was common practice (Cassidy, 2006; Selin and Stone, 2009), for example, amongst Australian Aboriginal and Torress Strait women (Kildea and Wardaguga, 2009).

As belief systems changed in Western and Middle Eastern thinking, persecution and control of women and midwives grew. Western culture became influenced by Christianity and Goddess worship vanished as more organised religion took root within communities. The Goddess spirituality became a domestic affair with the dominant patriarchal religiosity dominating the public world. The dark ages descended upon Europe and midwives, and women's birth knowledge and experience went underground (Brodsky, 2008). Women represented sexuality that was of the devil representing abeyance to senses. Paradoxically, birth became progressively hidden and feared as Western society evolved. There is little evidence of how those attuned at the moment of birth at this time. However, it is known that moods of shame, punishment, and fear at birth percolated society in the dark ages in response to the cultural interpretation of the early Christian scriptures that influenced much of Europe.

Bible and birth

Biblical stories of birth often depict suffering. According to some interpretations the imagery is a powerful deterrent (Kalmanofsky, 2008). Kalmanofsky believes the horror and pain of birth was used by the Old Testament authors as a ploy to bring Israel back into God's favour. Kalmanofsky interprets biblical childbirth as a metaphor for crisis, symbolic of the plight of Israel as exposed, vulnerable and at a time of suffering. The imagery is certainly vivid. Birth as a metaphor for crisis and fear is arguably a mood that continues into much of contemporary western birthing culture and experience.

The Old Testament writings were by men as far as we know who, at that time, were probably excluded from birth. Bergmann (2008) examined texts taken from the Ancient Orient and the Old Testament and found women's voices were hidden. What was experienced and meaningful at birth in those times remains open to biblical hermeneutic exegetic[2] interpretation. It is clear however that western culture has been profoundly influenced by Judaic-Christian biblical doctrines. For example, the birth of Jesus is a celebrated nativity in Christian culture recorded in the New Testament. Yet even the birth of Jesus was surrounded by crisis, including where to birth and the social political tensions of the era.[3]

Historical author, Anita Diamant, attempts to address the silent voice of biblical women in her novel *The Red Tent* (1998). Diamant provides a voice to biblical women in which joy, sacredness as well as the potential for death and suffering at birth, is described. In her novel the world of birth is interpreted as a shared womanly experience not one of continuing crisis. Of course, the reality of women's birthing practices and reproduction in those early times in history can only be conjecture because little is actually documented about the context of women's lives in that epoch.

Fear of birth and magical women

In early times, fear of birth as unclean, taboo, and dangerous fuelled prejudiced notions about women and birth through history and cross culturally (Kirkham, 2007). For example, the fear of the mysteries in and around birth induced stigmata[4] (Murray, 2007). Murray highlights how aspects of women's religious culture were found to be threatening to Jewish religious leaders of the first century. Women during these times were often suppressed and feared for their reproductive knowledge and abilities. Birth as female and private had become mysterious and associated with magic as something that could not be controlled. Those attending births came under scrutiny.

Suppressing women and vilifying them helped establish the authority and truth of the suppressor. When the witch hunt holocaust swept across Europe many centuries later ignited by such prejudices, it resulted in the execution of thousands of women. Following the 1486 Hammer of Witches, midwives were regarded as the guiltiest of demonic practisers and summarily put to death for practising their craft. In many cultures, and through history, birth was often understood as paradoxically auspicious yet unclean and dangerous thus tarnishing birth attendants with the danger of performing unholy acts. Despite these attitudes, beliefs and prejudices, and stories about respect and honouring of the midwife also stretch back in time; for example, Aristotle's own mother [*c.*300 bc] was a respected and revered midwife.

In Medieval Europe women would gather and assist each other at the birth. The mood of attendants and their charges as they went about their silenced hidden work remained unseen. They were known as 'god-sibs' providing the physical and emotional support through a woman's travail (Kitzinger, 2011). The god-sibs included the mother's sisters, her mother, grandmother, neighbours, and friends. Often their role would extend to be a Godmother; an important role in medieval Europe when maternal death was high, and survival of the infant thus ensured. It can be construed that these god-sibs attuned in a particular way. It can be speculated that the atmosphere would have been supportive and jovial. Unfortunately, again, this nurturing group would be criticised.[5]

Women, though central to the birth process, were silenced in the world of men with stories of birth uttered solely amongst women. Any moment of joy at birth remained within the women's world. Yet co-existing with such joy there would have been the spectre of pain, suffering, and death.

Pain and joy

The paradoxical coexistence of pain and joy is common in birth narratives. Across cultures, birth is a significant rite of passage that involves pain and joy emerging through ritualised practices. Anthropologists studying cross cultural birth describe dichotomous notions: agony and happiness, bitter then sweet, more pain than thought possible, then more happiness than thought possible (Davis-Floyd and Cheyney, 2009; Selin and Stone, 2009; Callister and Khalaf, 2009). Callister and Khalaf gathered the following words that describe birth in cross cultural stories:

> ... scary, exciting, easy, peaceful, beautiful, incredible, amazing, really hard, spiritual, humbling, joyful, bittersweet, painful, overwhelming, wonderful, satisfying, worthwhile, hard work, exhausting, frightening, indescribable, love, caring, awe and amazement, brilliant, it's just like it has an aura about it, magic, miracle, happiness, fulfilling, unknown, exhilarating, difficult, stressful, and rewarding ... no word to express the experience ... it is more than special. It is a gift and a privilege that God gives to women ... an overwhelming feeling of responsibility that gushes over you....
>
> (2009: 35–36)

Such words seem timeless. Historically, birth has brushed near to death the world over as the Chad proverb goes "when a woman enters childbirth, she has one foot in the grave" (Kitzinger, 2011). In the novel *The Red Tent*, the angel of death lurks in the background at birth waiting to take either or both. Women prepare themselves with prayer and other spiritual practices, their lives precarious, all cognisant of other women who have died. As Zisken (2002: 94), a Judaic poet, simply illustrates, birth involves challenge:

> A new baby born
> Born last night
> Smelling of roses
> Coming through the thorn
> Into the
> Shining light

There was a knowing that the "thorn" needed to be traversed to experience the light of joy. There came a time when men were called increasingly to assist as the thorn became a crisis and the light of joy threatened.

Early men-midwives at birth

The history of others at birth and across cultures has become progressively conflictive over the last 200 years. Male involvement in birth has a chequered history (Brodsky, 2008). Prior to the advent of obstetricians, barber-surgeons who later became known as men-midwives would come to births when invited by women. They had limited skills and little or no physiology or anatomy knowledge, having no access to medical education. Despite this, seventeenth-century men came progressively into the birthing room to face crisis. These early men-midwives were segregated from the physician who continued to be regarded as superior in status. Obstetrics, as a speciality taught in medical schools, was to come a century later.

In the late nineteenth and early twentieth century, obstetricians were charged with not antagonising women during birth. Mood at birth remained intimate and female focused. It is plausible that the mood to which early obstetricians attuned at birth would have been significantly different to midwives and others. Men at birth attuned to the crisis they were called upon to attend. Relationships with the labouring birthing woman and her family was not essential. The call for medical help would have invoked fear because events would not have been unfolding well. For the most part, birth continued within a women's world, but the tide was changing.

In the 1800s the professionalisation of men at birth was evolving. The pursuit of modernity, in the guise of industrialisation, was gaining momentum. The rise of science and modernity was affecting all aspects of life in the mid-1800s and this was no less than the case in the colonies. For the most part birth remained in the domain of women for European women settlers across the Americas and antipodeans. The world of midwifery and birth was also sustained by women in early colonists regions, even when the early men-midwives and obstetricians were called to birth (Ulrich, 1991; Clarke, 2012), whilst midwives and 'god-sibs' only called upon doctors in times of difficulty (Brodsky, 2008).

Death and birth were closely related in society and both kept discreet by early European colonists around the world. Social and geographical isolation, fear of death and suffering would have been a reality. Lack of sanitation, medical assistance and lack of extended family support would have made life hard, especially for the poor. Coupled with this was the socially constructed shame and distaste of anything sexual in Victorian society that permeated across much of European culture. Mere mention of the birthing process was distasteful. This need to conceal birth would have made birth a particularly trying time for European women, especially so for early European settlers in the colonies who found themselves amidst very different local birth cultures and far from their own families.

Indigenous birth cultures and colonisation

In nineteenth-century New Zealand (NZ), when colonisation began in earnest, Māori birth outcomes were scarcely acknowledged. Māori society and birthing practices were vastly different to the colonists.[6] The cosmology and community structure were also different. The once sacred nature and simplicity of Māori birthing changed as colonisation increased. The notion of Atua – central to birth as to all other aspects of life – recognises and honours the Tapu (restricting/sacred) and the Noa (common) essences of experiences and things: "Europeans could be ignorant or insensitive about Māori cultural practice, acting in ways that risked the spiritual and psychological well-being of the Whanau" (Clarke, 2012: 28). Both Māori and Pakeha, having survived a brush with death, would have undoubtedly been relieved. Clarke's (2012) maternity history of nineteenth century NZ recognises the bicultural birth experience of Māori and Pakeha women highlighting this commonality:

> The tales of two very different women, who represent two sides of this country's history, remind us that childbirth very often brought immense fulfilment and joy for those involved.
>
> (243)

For early NZ settlers and local indigenous people, culture was bound up with the natural process of birth and the joy at birth was a shared cross-cultural experience.

Ultrich's (1991) *Midwife's Tale* examines American seventeenth-century midwife Martha Ballad's diaries, highlighting the type of relationship that early colonist midwives had with mothers; a connection that appears congenial and emotionally enhancing. Familiarity of women-midwives with mothers was acknowledged and respected in contrast to the male doctor who would not have the same manner of emotional connection "… the word 'friends' appears repeatedly in doctor's writings from the mid-eighteenth to mid-nineteenth century … female healers identified with the patients they serve in ways that male physicians could not…" (ibid., 65). In the eighteenth and nineteenth century midwives and doctors were often found in acrimonious disputes where the growing men-midwives, who came to be known as obstetricians, were increasingly present at birth. Power struggles arose in the birthing room.

Popular fiction

As attendance of others at birth changed so too popular fiction contributed to views of changing moods at birth. Riley (1968) takes the reader on a disquieting and harrowing voyage through the literature in which birth is continually interpreted as bleak and cynical. There are only infrequent hints in the fictional classics of birth as something more than pain, death, and suffering requiring women to surrender and hope for survival. Yet something elusive is glimpsed occasionally in literature. Thackeray's novel, *Vanity Fair*, provides a glimpse of miracle at hearing the first cry of a baby yet avoids explicit descriptions about birth (Thackeray and Pollard, 1847/1978). This avoidance in the popular literature of the times only increased fear and mistrust.

The reputation of midwives and doctors at birth in the 1800s inspired authors to incite further anxiety and prejudice. The Dickensian novel, *Martin Chuzzlewit*,[7] paints Mrs Sairy Gamp, a community midwife, as uncaring, uneducated, lacking integrity, callous, and frequently drunk. Dickens also criticised the conditions of birth and the men-midwives of the time in *Little Dorrit*.[8] Without doubt the physical and social conditions of nineteenth-century maternity for most people in the UK would have generally been unpleasant and needed to be exposed. Although birth appears cloaked in cultural prejudices across time, something beyond the physical event of birth remained silenced.

Women would have had to find information and help where they could because little written information about birth was accessible. However, the following excerpt from a late 1800's book called *Tokology* points towards something more at birth:

> What more helpless and dependent than the newborn infant! A human soul, with all the possibilities of life, yet of itself it cannot supply its slightest need. No wonder that so great a wealth of maternal love is called forth in administering to such helplessness! No wonder that the mother's heart is humbled at the greatness of her mission as special guardian of the little one! May divine love and wisdom aid and guide her!
>
> (Stockham, 1890: 204)

Perhaps this was an 1890s challenge to the increasing obstetric presence at births and the perennial lack of skilled assistance. There was resistance to educating midwives in the western world and colonies and a growing focus on birth as pathological. De Lee, an American obstetrician, argued that birth was pathological, promoted prophylactic forceps deliveries, and campaigned in the early 1900s against midwifery (Murphy-Lawless, 1998). Most western nations were similarly organising maternity care and the attunement at birth gradually changed to something public and less personal (For example, in 1902 the UK midwives act came into being, outlawing untrained or lay midwives from practice. Likewise, in 1925, the New Zealand Nurses and Midwives Registration Act ended the legitimate practice of untrained handy-woman birth attendants). Although this would appear good news, it coincided with how industrialisation was entering the birth space and was the harbinger of control and increasing structural organisation around birth.

Infant Sorrow

My mother groan'd! my father wept.
Into the dangerous world I leapt:
Helpless, naked, piping loud:
Like a fiend hid in a cloud.
Struggling in my father's hands,
Striving against my swaddling bands,
Bound and weary I thought best
To sulk upon my mother's breast.
        (William Blake 1757–1827)

Blake's poem criticises the wave of industrialisation in the eighteenth and nineteenth century. The symbolism illustrates the anguish of birth and a future endured in the world of depersonalised modernity. Even the nurture of suckling is denied in this new world as Blake helplessly surrenders to destiny sulking at his mother's breast. Industrialisation brought an era attuned to scientific reasoning when aspects of life had mere utility value. It ushered political change in the guise of liberal democracy and social reform. The poem evokes a sense of birth as a social mechanism to feed the industrial cogs of the new thinking. Any joy would seem hidden in the avalanche of modernity's vicissitudes.

Technology era

Obstetrician

The evolution of technology was an aspect of the increasing presence of the new birth professional; the specialist obstetrician. Yet the position of obstetricians has not been easy. They were, and still are, only called in NZ and the UK when things are not going well. In the early days of obstetrics there was little that could be done for haemorrhage, pain, infection, and eclampsia. Ergot preparations were used for bleeding by herbalist midwives, but dosage was hard to calculate and often resulted in harm in the hands of the less skilled. Pharmacological utero-tonics did not appear until the twentieth century and death through haemorrhage continued to be the plight of many birthing women until such drug preparations were refined and available. Conversely, pharmaceutical pain relief was an early contribution welcomed by many and changed the way many attuned at birth in dramatic ways.

Evolution of pain-free birth

The evolution of obstetric analgesia attuned birth in ways not previously experienced. This is dramatically illustrated in the emergence of 'twilight' birth. Chloroform, an early analgesic, was initially available only to the socially elite. Its use is depicted in Mackensie's 1912 novel, *Carnival,*[9] about a woman given chloroform towards the end of her labour who slips into oblivion awaking after to meet her newborn. This is not to infer woman had no choice. The diaries of women in early 1900s England depict the domestic nature of birth and highlight women's choice (Llewelyn Davis, 1915/1978). Twilight sleep births become progressively popular from 1914 after introduction in Germany where it was called Dammerschlaf. Twilight sleep was actively welcomed and had become common in New Zealand by the mid-1940s (Clarke, 2012). Mothers would be routinely anesthetised for the labour and birth and awake after the birth, as a New Zealand obstetrician in the early to mid-twentieth century describes:

> When the baby was four hours old, and Rose was out of her anaesthetic to appreciate the situation, I carried in the infant. 'Rose, I've got your baby here ... would you like to touch her wee hand?
>
> (Gordon, 1957: 64)

She then elaborates:

> One could never forget the little wife who, having disclosed to me her secret dread of labour pains, sampled my earlier twilight sleep technique and opened her mouth just after her babe was born to sing in a sweet treble, "I dreamt I walked with God in the garden!"
>
> (67)

The practice continued in New Zealand into the 1960s, and until the 1970s in the UK and USA, until the introduction of epidurals. Other analgesic injections and inhalants were developed through the twentieth century. Eventually epidurals and the new obstetric anaesthetist arrived in the latter part of the twentieth century. Such advances were welcomed and continue to be requested to ease the pain of birth thus further shaping the birth experience for many women around the world, for example, in New Zealand (McAra-Couper *et al.*, 2012; Douche, 2009) and Canada (Stoll and Hall, 2013). How society attunes to birth has become progressively positioned in a technology. Although, a recent review of the literature has shown that what matters to women overall is a positive birth experience that acknowledges and attends to their psychosocial needs too (Downe *et al.*, 2018).

Any discussion on birth would not be complete without recognition of death that can and does arrive at birth on occasions; either the woman's death or that of her infant(s), or both.

Maternal death

Obstetricians, both past and present, are charged with reducing maternal death and morbidity and thus are placed in an unenviable position. Obstetricians in the nineteenth and early twentieth century would have had little at their disposal to save lives. Deaths attributed to eclampsia and infection continued. Eclampsia remained untreatable and women frequently died well into the twentieth century.

A dramatic depiction of death in 1920 from eclampsia illustrates the helplessness of the obstetrician and local GP in a British period drama set within post-Edwardian England *Downton Abbey* (Webb and Fellowes, 2012). After an aristocratic homebirth, the mother begins fitting. The medical men essentially stood back helpless as she convulsed and died; the grief-stricken father stood in the corner of the room holding the newborn. It was not only those in poverty that continued to suffer and die. The grandmother in this Downton Abbey story poignantly comments that "... mothers die and sad as that is, it is a part of life". The mood in the household, both in the family and the servant quarters, was despairing at the loss of the mother yet there was also a glimpse of happiness for the surviving newborn. In some tragic situations both mother and baby would die. Yet as birth came progressively under the auspices of medicine, another spectre of misfortune struck. As interventions and increasing hospital bed provision occurred, maternal death increased. Any joy at birth would have been juxtaposed with the increasing fear of death and suffering as women began increasingly to birth in institutions.

Although the early to mid-twentieth century was regarded as the golden age of medicine, a major risk of this time was death by iatrogenic puerperal sepsis (post-birth infection) and the terror of maternal mortality worsened. Coinciding with an increase in hospital birth, rates of maternal death due to sepsis increased. From early times, infection continued to prove difficult for the emerging new science of obstetrics. Conflict over what was to be seen as 'meddlesome' midwifery (obstetric interventions such as instrumental births) and fiscal issues endured through the interwar years. Despite this, hospital-based medicine started to gain respect as techniques for asepsis (keeping birth clean), introduction of antiseptics, and reducing mixed hospital wards brought infections down. The introduction of sulphonamides in the late 1930s, and antibiotics in 1945, further reduced the human misery of sepsis making hospital birth safer than before. However, the mood of childbirth had changed and became less attuned to social and domestic concerns and entered an era of public births.

Domestic to public

Maternity through cultures and history is one of following fads and trends. One of these pertains to the place to birth. In some cultures, birth occurred in dwellings separate from the home (Stone, 2009), examples of which could be found in India (Naraindas, 2009), New Zealand Māori (Rimene *et al.*, 1998) and Japan (Yanagisawa, 2009). Having birthing separate from domestic living quarters is connected to ideas of birth as polluting and due to beliefs concerned with attracting evil spirits and misfortune (Begay, 2009; Kitzinger, 2012; Dureau, 2009). In some cultures, birthing occurred outside or in specially constructed dwellings (Cassidy, 2006). First peoples and indigenous peoples birthing practices and birthing outside was vastly different to nineteenth century Europeans and European colonists who, for the most part, birthed at home on a bed.

Perhaps bizarrely for us now is how the early maternity hospitals were stigmatised as places for the destitute and women of low morals. They were dirty, overcrowded and places where the early men-midwives/obstetricians could experiment and learn. Infections and death rates were high; they were unpopular places to birth. The first maternity hospitals were opened in the 1800s and by 1940 there were over 1000 maternity beds within maternity hospitals across the UK alone. The journey from domestic to public in western culture had started and hospitals began increasingly to centralise and relocate the place of birth across much of the western world. As this occurred, women had progressively less say on the maternity care they received. Midwives lost their autonomy and birth became centralised, state organised, and medically controlled (Pairman, 2010). Birth had become institutionalised and procedural. By the mid-1930s western hospital birth under the supervision of a doctor was viewed as safe and became expected and desirable.

As this massive birth culture change took hold 'something' about the Being-with relationship at birth became hidden in the move to public institutions. The domestic private womanly process was now institutionally separate from communities. Maternity services were medical, and male dominated with midwives working as assistants. Place of birth had changed significantly in a short period of time and brought changes to mood at birth. A change in the authority of who was at birth and where birth happened had occurred – not everyone was happy with the changes and the language of maternity care history, as Tania McIntosh (2012) examination of the social history of childbirth revealed, it was akin to a military battle for control for power and financial gain.

Many parts of the western world in the 1980s and 90s witnessed political challenges and grassroots activism to maintain homebirth services for those that wanted to avoid hospitalisation. Such activism started to appear across western countries and westernised colonies. Today, place of birth remains a persistently disputed topic that can seem like a battle between opposing research agendas (Crowther *et al.*, 2010; Zielinski *et al.*, 2015; Grünebaum *et al.*, 2015). The mood at birth in such dichotomous positioning risks becoming covered over as we find ourselves increasingly fallen into a discourse on one side or the other; a discourse formed by the industrial revolution and the increasing dominance of medicalisation.

Industrialisation and medicalisation

Institutionalisation was a by-product of an era that had begun back in the late 1700s. The notions of industrialised and medicalised births have subtle yet significant differences. Medicalisation is employed to improve outcomes, whilst industrialised birth is more about standardisation, control, and centralisation. The industrial model, keen to maintain economic control over something unpredictable, promoted technocratic medicalised birthing practices. This became a confrontational rhetoric in the late twentieth century that continues today. Michel Odent (2001) argued two decades ago that the industrialisation of society mirrors the industrialisation of human birth; a story of controlling and disturbing. Perhaps not much has changed? There continues to be dissonance between medicalisation as overly technocratic but at the same time providing lifesaving possibilities. What is evident is that it is not necessarily the medicalisation that is at issue but the industrial context in which it is used.

Throughout the past 100 years the mood of midwifery texts has changed and increasingly favoured the scientific model of care which privileges medical technology. Early midwifery texts were very procedural. For example, Corkill's (1932) manual of management conforming to the syllabus of the Nurses and Midwives Registration Board in New Zealand contains no mention of relationships or the emotional or spiritual aspects of birth. This is perhaps a reflection on a time when many women and babies continued to die.

Not all obstetricians attuned to the industrial and medicalised model of childbirth. Grantly Dick Read [1890–1959] resisted and challenged the degree of interference at birth. He believed birth should be calm and peaceful. Fear, he suggested, was the enemy of natural birth. *Natural Childbirth* (1933) and *Childbirth Without Fear* (1942) became internationally recognised as proclaiming a new approach to obstetric practice. Dick-Read condemned much of the media fear-inducing propaganda. He especially scorned novelists for dramatising the fear of birth. He drew attention to how birth was attuned and encouraged an awakening of mood other than fear. He was criticised by professional contemporaries but celebrated by women who were at the time challenging the birth practices they were experiencing. His books were published at a time of rapid change in perception about birth. The desire to replace the unpredictable with the predicable gained favour. The 1950s, for example, heralded the development of antenatal care and an increasing focus on the physical wellbeing of the foetus.

Antenatal care and focus on the baby

The proliferation of antenatal care in the twentieth century saw the increasing medicalisation of reproduction. From the 1950s, biopolitics shifted focus to the unborn baby (Weir, 2006). The foetus increasingly occupied a central concern in maternity care and the sociological evolution of birth altered how many western countries attuned to reproduction. At the same time maternity services became increasingly technocratic, structured, and standardised in order to improve certain outcomes. The move from domestic and private to the public sphere had taken place, and a new approach to childbirth emerged comprising improved living conditions, less painful labour and births, and new reproductive technologies reducing perinatal deaths. An evolution from social to technocratic childbirth was taking place.

Evolution from social to technocratic

The evolution of technology and increasing medicalisation of birth replaced the social model of birthing that had existed for a millennium (Davis-Floyd, 2017). The trend continued with minimal opposition. From the 1950s, the community intimate focus diminished and the overall way of attuning to birth appeared more fearful despite improvements in outcomes. The focus was on avoiding risk and danger. Notions of sacred or spiritual birth had little place in this new world. Yet there were still those who condemned the technological positioning of birth.

Lamaze, a French obstetrician, focused on pain free labour and birth. The magic and mystery of a natural physiological birth attuned him towards something more than the procedural aspects of birth in the mid-twentieth century. His book *Painless Childbirth; the Lamaze method* was published in the middle of the twentieth century and hints at preserving the 'specialness' inherent at birth (Lamaze, 1956). However, many practitioners continued to embrace technology because it seemed to reduce the uncertainties associated with birth. The concept of birth as normal was only accepted retrospectively. Suzanne Arms (1996) suggests that, by the 1970s, technology had gone too far in its pursuit of rescuing from the expected dangers inherent in the birth process. She claims that the whole maternity system was built on fear and the expectation of pathology. This supports De Lee's 1900 pronouncements of childbirth as dangerous and in need of medical management in his publication *The De Lee protocols – The Pathologization*[10] *of Childbirth*. Scientism had fully invaded the birthing room and by 1955 95 per cent of women in the USA were birthing in institutions having medically managed births. A mood of seeking out problems rather than promoting the natural physiological process prevailed. The western medical model of maternity care gained increasing authority at birth and women became passive recipients of that care.

The polemic discourse of abnormal/pathological versus normal/natural fuelled a culture of risk management and mistrust in the physiological process provoking debate (Byrom and Downe, 2015; Chadwick and Foster, 2014; Scamell, 2014; Bryers and Van Teijlingen, 2010). The specialness of birth became hidden in pursuit of the scientifically managed birth. Yet it is also possible that the concern of society to protect birth by controlling and making it predictable could be due to birth's specialness beyond bio-medical concerns. Although this came with its own risk, it would seem that society's concern for birth safety had paradoxically hidden its specialness.

Birth as a social occasion became replaced by something under the public gaze and separated from community. The rhythms of labour and birth began to be replaced by timings and structured labours and births that followed defined parameters or required intervention. A commonly used textbook for UK midwives reflects the technical and procedurally focussed practice in the 1970s:

> It is inevitable in this mechanised age that the seventh edition has technological bias ... new photographs depict some aspects in which mechanical aids are being employed.
>
> (Myles, 1971: vii)

The pictures in this 1971 textbook depict midwives and doctors clad in white gowns adorned with masks in a clinical institutional environment. The woman having a baby is clearly in the role of 'patient'. The instruction to the midwife at the moment of birth is to look at the clock so that the exact time can be recorded on the birth certificate. This UK text mirrors the New Zealand medical obstetric text written at the time (Green, 1970). A demeanour of detachment to birth permeates these instructional manuals. A midwife's poem of the same era challenges the detached nature of medical presence:

> Procedure-normal spontaneous delivery.
> He couldn't have been with her.
> He couldn't have marvelled as she reached down,
> Drawing her daughter to her breast
> Laughing, shouting, crying- all the emotions of birth.
> No, he couldn't have been with her.
>
> (*The Essence of Midwifery* by Walsh.
> In: Styles and Moccia, 1993: 198–199)

This poem hints at the mood attuned to at this birth and reflects the beginning of a groundswell of feminism. However, it would be decades and a second wave of feminism in the 70s and 80s before women's and midwives' voices would begin to be heard.

Mood at birth begins to be reawakened

Ina May Gaskin, an American midwife, who worked to revitalise American midwifery, promoting sensitive approaches to birth began to publish in the early 1970s. Her seminal book, *Spiritual Midwifery*, published in 1977 has undergone several editions. She continues to advocate that birth is sacred and the experience is special for all involved (Gaskin, 1977, 2011). Her focus is on gentle, women-centred midwifery practice enacted safely in the 'right' state of mind. Gaskin points to an attuned way at birth that encompasses more than the medicalisation prevailing at the time.

Another book written in the early 70s is by Frédérick Leboyer, who gestures to a moment attuned to a particular mood at birth:

> Birth may be a matter of a moment. But it is a unique one. To be born means to begin to breathe, to embark on that perpetual motion which will be with us till we die.
>
> (Leboyer, 1991: 99)

This excerpt from *Birth without Violence* hints at how birth projects into future possibilities. Leboyer raised awareness of the newborn and the manner in which a baby is introduced to the world. The moment of birth was acknowledged as significant. Bringing birth to awareness rather than blindly following social constructions of birth is congruent with Heidegger's notion of authenticity and not being swayed by the One's (The They) prescriptive approach to birth.

With the twists and turns of each epoch and popular trends midwifery has found itself attuning to the prevailing mood of the times. Textbooks, medical audits, statistics, and reductionist research methodologies continued to prove the validity of technocratic births into the twenty-first century. The growth of mass media has also influenced acceptance of technology in the name of safety and pain free birthing. This is a trend epitomised by the rise and the normalisation of caesarean sections. The euphemism of the 'natural caesarean' used by the media drew public attention in London in the 1990s and 2000s as a woman-centred approach to birth (Smith *et al.*, 2008). The increasing use and demand by women for birth technology seemed to act as catalyst for the further proliferation of technological intervention. Throughout these changes the quiet voice that pleads for women to be seen, heard, involved and placed at the centre of childbirth continually whispered, albeit often silenced in the early days, a whisper that consistently yearned for tenderness amongst the moods of social political change.

Feminism and birth

Feminism is not a homogenous ideology. The first wave of feminists in the nineteenth and early twentieth century focused on suffrage and overturning legal obstacles with little focus on the reproductive rights of women. In the mid-twentieth century feminism was to take another turn. Simone de Beauvoir, a feminist philosopher, was concerned that women were being perceived as "other" in the patriarchal society. She concluded that male-centred ideology served to reinforce the notion that women are different due to their capacity to birth. This was not a rationale, she argued, for positioning them as an inferior gender (de Beauvoir, 1949/2009). Her book *The Second Sex* was influential in igniting the second wave of feminism; a wave of feminism that focused on inequality issues such as reproductive rights and family planning. With the advent of contraception and the second wave of feminism in the late 60s and early 70s women had fewer babies. Choice and control over the experience of birth began to be sought as the feminist movement gained momentum in the 1960s and 1970s. Although survival remains central to safe care, it was addressing the experience of birth which became increasingly a feminist issue.

The second wave of feminism highlighted the dissonance in the western phenomenon of birth; being safe versus wanting individualised care that lessened medical interference. Women argued that it was not either safety or positive experience they sought – it was both. Notwithstanding the heated debates in feminist literature, birth as a significant social event extended beyond feminist concerns (Crouch and Manderson, 1993). The socio-political mood of many western maternity cultures in the 1970s and 80s was confrontational and volatile.

The mood was changing, and feminism was evolving. A third wave of feminism from the late 1980s and early 1990s onwards, often co-existing with the second wave notions, addressed diversity and cultural differences (Tong, 2009). Midwifery and maternity care in the second and third waves of feminism became a central feminist issue leading to social change in maternity care provision. The third wave of feminism increasingly emphasised the desire for consensus decision-making with women at the centre. Being actively aware, having choices over the birth process, and positive experiences increasingly gained popularity in the 1980s.

During these turbulent years there was evidence of gentle affirming care that acknowledged the unique specialness at birth (Balaskas, 1989; Bowen, 1993/2000). In the 1980s, UK obstetrician Wendy Savage emphasised individualised care and won wide support at the time. An advocate for change in the UK, she called for an end to the controlling nature of obstetrics (Savage, 1986). The voices of women emerged more clearly in political discourse. Hierarchical organisation of maternity care was not acceptable in the new feminist discourse. The third wave of feminism, akin to post-structuralism, focused on the individual as unique. As the focus of feminism unfolded so did further emphasis on birth experience.

Apogee of 'good birth'

Obstetric hegemony was challenged at the end of the 60s through to the 80s. The fight for choice and empowerment of women became increasingly visible. The experience of birth was also becoming more central. Something special at birth was beginning to be recognised and sought. A London based obstetrician states: "Modern-day life and our highly stressed, risk adverse societies have led to medicalised, fearful model of childbirth, which has stripped the process of its wondrous magic" (Lokugamage, 2011: 78). It was as if the mood of wonder or joy at birth called to be reawakened. The hint of magic at birth resonated in the desire for reaching the apogee or peak of birth experience. The search was on for "... an exalted quality of the birth experience that represents an existential moment in women's lives" (Crouch and Manderson, 1993:56). The political ramifications reverberated globally in the western community.

Fathers and intimate others welcomed at birth

Part of this emerging choice and control related to who could be present at birth. This was a time of emerging parental rights as an extension of feminist rights; the baby was now "our baby". In the western context, fathers' presence at birth began gradually from the early 1960s (Mander, 2004). They were invited by their partners in the belief that the presence of a familiar other would alleviate anxiety in the alien medical world. In addition, there was the assumption that the presence at the birth would facilitate attachment with the newborn and strengthen marital relationships. Yet fathers have, on occasions, been at birth throughout history and within some traditional cultures such as found in Tibet (Craig, 2009). Māori men have also acted as midwives and supporters (Clarke, 2012). In European homes, fathers were often present to help and take on tasks given to them by the midwife.

Today there is an expectation that partners (fathers and same sex partners) participate and it is unusual to attend a birth in the western context when the partner of the woman is not present. What is evident is that men had become part of the birth environment, either as health care professional or family or friend. Not everyone was happy with men in the birthing room. Some believe the introduction of the father to the labour and birth is disruptive and detrimental to the physiological process (Odent, 2002). As with all changes and new trends, the debate continues. In this age of choice and the importance of positive experience it is hard to imagine that a partner would be denied access to 'being-there' in the room physically, if that is the choice of the women and the partner wants to be there. However, how partners gather and attune collectively with others at birth, how they are affected, and what it means to them remains mainly hidden. This could merely be another fashionable social practice in the evolution of human birth.

The political struggles and tension between society's wish for improved experiences have been coupled with publicised medical mishaps and choice violations. What is emerging is the central desire for the maternity experience to be relational. Over time trusting relationships in the maternity system are being sought (Lewis *et al.*, 2017). There is a growing desire for individualised positive experiences and relational continuity across the childbirth experience. The evidence for continuity of care from a midwife continues to emerge along with increasing knowledge on how to enact and sustain this model of care provision (Sandall *et al.*, 2016; Homer *et al.*, 2019; Gilkison *et al.*, 2015).

Returning to relationships

Modern day western midwifery now speaks progressively more and more in terms of partnership, openness, flexibility, and collaboration with women without compromising safety. Such a partnership model embraces feminist issues of power and liberation of women from the tyranny of hegemonic patriarchal medicine; it is a model based on relationships. These emerging cultural values engender autonomous and empowered midwifery supported by the requests from women and their families. As Lesley Page (1995) stated back in the mid-90s the focus of maternity is not about working on women but with women. The new focus avoids 'jumping in' to do things but provides the opportunity for the birth to unfold with minimal interference (Smythe, 2010). Partnership thus invokes a sense of reciprocity and equality, of something shared (Kirkham, 2010) avoiding authoritarian coercive modes of communicating (Pairman, 2010) seeking a shared commitment to optimal birth experiences that both families and midwives enjoy (Smythe *et al.*, 2014). Acknowledging the importance of returning to relationships in and around childbirth re-attunes the mood and subsequent experience. However, this return to a need and desire for positive relational care is juxtaposed to the messages of mass media which continues to influence the mood of contemporary birth.

Media attunement

Popular TV sitcoms often depict women screaming for help as they are safely delivered in the hands of the hospital staff. *Call the Midwife* and *One Born Every Minute*, two UK based television dramas broadcast in many global regions, depict birth in a variety of often dramatic scenes. Both focus on the dramatic spectacle of childbirth. Yet *Call the Midwife*, the original autobiography of a midwife in post-war 1950s East London slums, also clearly depicts the joy and awe of birth amidst social-economic deprivation:

> …I am almost as overwhelmed as Muriel; the relief of a safe delivery is so powerful…. He breathes. The baby is now a separate being. I wrap him in towels given to me, and hand him to Muriel, who cradles him, coos over him, kisses him, calls him "beautiful, lovely, an angel".
>
> (Worth, 2002: 11–12)

Conversely, televised and film depictions can fuel a fear culture. The simple miracle of birth can become hidden in the miracles of modern science that saves and protects. Stories of drama and anxious moments dominate the narratives often leaving the moment of joy at birth concealed as illustrated in this field note:

> Student midwives in a tutorial explained to me how the mood of twenty-first century birth in their experience was one of fear. Yet juxtaposed to this fear culture is the joy in the same student's faces as they tell of the moment at birth itself.
>
> (Field notes, 2012)

Contemporary birth mythology

There is a modern western birth mythology; the drama is in the emergency caesarean section, the heated and anxious moments within an instrumental birth, the haemorrhaging woman, and the ambulance transfer to a major hospital from a rural area. There is the sense of women's helplessness, of being thrown into motherhood, having to sacrifice herself completely; even if, in a western twenty-first century maternity hospital, she is unlikely to make the ultimate sacrifice of death for her baby(s). It would seem that, despite the renewed maternity mood being revealed, many birth attendants and partners continue to be attuned to fear of birth yet at the same time are affected by the specialness at birth. It is clear that control and aversion to anything less than perfect outcomes dominate practice and experience so that technological birth cannot be refused or rejected. On the contrary, much technology around childbirth is often welcomed by families and maternity care providers alike in contemporary western maternity (McAra-Couper *et al.*, 2010). What is curious is that this does not lesson fear around childbirth. Some would even argue that the fear of birth as a result of technology attunes birth to more fear. Whilst the notion of what constitutes a 'good birth' continues to be unpacked (Smythe *et al.*, 2016), a newly attuned mythology has emerged. The real *fear* is perhaps related to uneasiness with *what* has been hidden. I would contend that within the birth experience something hints at the spirit of birth risks being lost.

Conclusion

The story of birth is a human journey of mysterious beginnings, a story that is connected with creation and evolution that is culturally and socially constructed. I have accessed resources specifically to respond to hermeneutic questions and concede that not all aspects of such a complex phenomenon can be addressed. I acknowledge that alongside my selection and interpretation I privilege certain perspectives which touch and call to me. The aim of this chapter is to fore-ground the complexity of our human birthing story and attune the reader to the vast phenomenon of childbirth, not present the whole story of human birth – indeed that would not be possible!

This chapter has shown how twenty-first century maternity manifests change and a sense of hope. Yet, at the same time gestures to something conspicuously absent in the language of birth that weaves itself through history. Here we live in the early part of the twenty-first century surveying many aspects of childbirth, yet we could be passing over and eliding something important at birth. It is not a story that can be completed, there is much still to be revealed. For me, the phenomenon of joy at birth is what concerns and beckons my thinking. Joy at birth is an attunement that is often relegated to a passing comment or paragraph at the most, sometimes a mere inference for the reader to ponder. But what is this joy, how is it there, what is its meaning? How is it experienced? When it is absent, covered over or hidden what does that signify? I remain curious to know. Does joy at birth gift something of significance that reveals the spirit of birth? Does joy at birth gesture to existential meaning for us all? I would maintain that the experience and meaning of such a mood in and around birth remains fundamentally unspoken.

Mysterious holy voyage
Women's magic –
Thorny
hidden and sacred
silenced
uncertain
yet
When we industrialise -
how do we attune?
Centralised and standardised –
how do we attune?
Medicalised,
become technocratic, electric and mechanised–
how do we attune?
Globalisation and consumerism –
neo-colonialism
new feminism
how do we attune?
–
A baby born –
into the light
alive, unfurling
we are silenced
how do we attune?

(Field notes, 2012)

Notes

1 Altricial is an inability to self-care at birth, in contrast to precocial species that are relatively mature and mobile from the moment of birth. Precocial species are those in which the young are relatively mature and mobile from the moment of birth.
2 Exegesis: Refers to critical interpretation of a text by attempting to determine historical context, such as when examining religious scripture.
3 I am aware that care is required in comparing the birth of Jesus with other births. Jesus's birth was a holy event for many. What is being revealed here is that the birth of avatars, saints, and prophets are often depicted as both challenge and joyous hope. The symbolism provides a powerful indication of the power of birth and its possibilities. It can be imagined that the birth of Jesus was fearful and full of hope. The actual lived-experience of Mary and Joseph at the moment of birth however is not revealed.
4 Stigmata is a mark of disgrace associated with a particular circumstance, such as birth and being a woman. It is also part of Christian traditional beliefs in which physical marks/wounds appear that correspond to those left on Christ's body by the Crucifixion, including bleeding from hands and feet.

5 The term 'god-sib' etymologically evolved to 'gossips' which later became a negative description of women speaking together (Kitzinger, 2011).
6 Any reading on Māori culture is my own interpretation. From my understanding there are two broad main differences in worldview; a western individualism that was juxtaposed to the Māori collective living which is more interconnected and less hegemonic with a spirit-world consciousness that informs Māori Tikanga (values/customs and rules). The intention is not to delve into Māori beliefs as I am not Māori. I came to NZ in 2005 in my mid 40s and have not been immersed in Māoritanga (Maori culture). Although I have taken te reo Māori (Māori language) classes and cultural safety seminars, I remain largely naïve about Māori culture and history.
7 Dickens, C. (1844). *Martin Chuzzlewit*. Chapman & Hall.
8 See the Charles Dicken's novel *Little Dorrit* published in 1857.
9 Mackenzie, C. (2012). *Carnival*. London: Floating Press.
10 For an overview and social critique of DeLee's work see Lewis, C.H. (2015). The gospel of good obstetrics: Joseph Bolivar DeLee's vision for childbirth in the United States. *Social History of Medicine*, 29(1), pp. 112–130.

References

Arms, S. (1996). *Immaculate Deception 11: Myth, Magic & Birth*. Berkeley, CA: Celestial Arts.

Balaskas, J. (1989). *New Active Birth; A Concise Guide to Natural Childbirth*. London: Unwin.

Begay, R.C. (2009). Navajo birth: A bridge between the past and the future. In: H. Selin and P.K. Stone, eds, *Childbirth across Cultures: Ideas and Practices of Pregnancy, Childbirth and the Postpartum*, New York: Springer, pp. 245–251.

Bergmann, C.D. (2008). *Childbirth as a Metaphor for Crisis: Evidence from the Ancient Near East, the Hebrew Bible and IQHXI, 1–18*. New York: Walter de Gmyter.

Bowen, S. (1993/2000). A midwife's prayer. In: L.P. Hunter, ed., *Birthwork*. La Jolla, CA: Pacifica Editions Publisher, pp. 4–6.

Brodsky, P.L. (2008). *The Control of Childbirth*. London: McFarland & Company, Inc., Publishers.

Bryers, H.M. and Van Teijlingen, E. (2010). Risk, theory, social and medical models: A critical analysis of the concept of risk in maternity care. *Midwifery*, 26, pp. 488–496.

Byrom, S. and Downe, S. (2015). *The Roar behind the Silence: Why Kindness, Compassion and Respect Matter in Maternity Care*. London: Pinter & Martin.

Callister, L.C. and Khalaf, I. (2009). Culturally diverse women giving birth: Their stories. In: H. Selin and P.K. Stone, eds, *Childbirth across Cultures: Ideas and Practices of Pregnancy, Childbirth and the Postpartum*. New York: Springer, pp. 33–40.

Callister, L.C. and Khalaf, I. (2010). Spirituality in childbearing women. *Journal of Perinatal Education*, 19, pp. 16–24.

Campanelli, P. and Campanelli, D. (1998). *Pagan Rites of Passage*. St Paul, MN: Llewellyn Publications.

Cassidy, T. (2006). *Birth: The Surprising History of How We Are Born*. New York: Atlantic Monthly Press.

Chadwick, R.J. and Foster, D. (2014). Negotiating risky bodies: Childbirth and constructions of risk. *Health, Risk & Society*, 16, pp. 68–83.

Clarke, A. (2012). *Born to a Changing World*. Wellington, NZ: Bridget Williams Books.

Corkill, T.F. (1932). *Lectures on Midwifery and Infant Care; a New Zealand Course*. Auckland, NZ: Coullis Somerville Wilke Ltd.

Craig, S.R. (2009). Pregnancy and childbirth in Tibet: Knowledge, perspectives, and practices. In: H. Selin and P.K. Stone, eds, *Childbirth across Cultures: Ideas and Practices of Pregnancy, Childbirth and the Postpartum*. New York: Springer, pp. 145–160.

Crouch, M. and Manderson, L. (1993). Parturition as social metaphor. *The Australian and New Zealand Journal of Sociology*, 29, pp. 55–72.

Crowley, V. (2001). *A Women's Guide to the Earth Traditions*. London: Thorsons.

Crowther, S., Gilkison, A., and Hunter, M. (2010). Comment on the Wax *et al.*, (2010). Meta-analysis of home vs. hospital birth. *New Zealand College of Midwives Journal*, pp. 19–21.

Davis-Floyd, R. (2017). *Ways of Knowing about Birth: Mothers, Midwives, Medicine, and Birth Activism*. Long Grove, IL: Waveland Press.

Davis-Floyd, R. and Cheyney, M. (2009). Birth and the big bad wolf: An evolutionary perspective. In: H. Selin and P.K. Stone, ed., *Childbirth across Cultures: Ideas and Practices of Pregnancy, Childbirth and the Postpartum*. New York: Springer, pp. 1–22.

de Beauvoir, S. (1949/2009). *The Second Sex*. London: Random House.

Delaporte, M. and Martin, M. (2018). *Sacred Inception: Reclaiming the Spirituality of Birth in the Modern World*. Lanham, MD: Lexington Books.

Diamant, A. (1998). *The Red Tent*. Crows Nest, Australia: Allen and Unwin.

Dick-Read, G. (1933). *Natural Childbirth*. London: William Heinemann (Medical Books) Limited.

Dick-Read, G. (1942). *Childbirth without Fear: The Principles and Practice of Natural Childbirth*. London: Heinemann Medical Books.

Douche, J. (2009). Rhetorical (de)vices and the construction of a 'natural' caesarian. *New Zealand College of Midwives Journal*, 40, pp. 20–23.

Downe, S., Finlayson, K., Oladapo, O., Bonet, M., and Metin Gülmezoglu, A. (2018). What matters to women during childbirth: A systematic qualitative review. *PloS One*, 13, p. e0194906.

Dureau, C. (2009). Converting birth in Simbo, Western Solomon Islands. In: H. Selin and P.K. Stone, eds, *Childbirth across Cultures: Ideas and Practices of Pregnancy, Childbirth and the Postpartum*. New York: Springer, pp. 265–274.

Gaskin, I.M. (1977). *Spiritual Midwifery*. Summertown, TN: The Book Publishing Company.

Gaskin, I.M. (2011). *Birth Matters – A Midwife's Manifesta*. New York: Seven Stories Press.

Gilkison, A., McAra-Couper, J., Gunn, J., *et al.* (2015). Midwifery practice arrangements which sustain case-loading Lead Maternity Carer midwives in New Zealand. *NZCOM Journal*, 51, pp. 11–16.

Gordon, D. (1957). *Doctor Down Under*. London: Faber & Faber.

Green, G.H. (1970). *Introduction to Obstetrics*. Christchurch, NZ: N.M. Pertyer Ltd.

Grünebaum, A., McCullough, L.B., Arabin, B., Brent, R.L., Levene, M.I., and Chervenak, F.A. (2015). Home birth is unsafe: FOR: The safety of planned homebirths: a clinical fiction. *BJOG: An International Journal of Obstetrics & Gynaecology*, 122, pp. 1235–1235.

Hanely, J. and Brown, A. (2014). Cultural variations in interpretation of postnatal illness: Jinn possession amongst Muslim communities. *Community Mental Health Journal*, 50, pp. 348–353.

Heidegger, M. (1927/1962). *Being and Time*. New York: Harper.

Hennessey, A.M. and Davis-Floyd, R.E. (2018). *Imagery, Ritual, and Birth: Ontology between the Sacred and the Secular*. Lanham, MD: Lexington Books.

Hill, K. (2011). *The God Revolution*. Auckland, NZ: Attar Books.

Holten, L. and de Miranda, E. (2016). Women's motivations for having unassisted childbirth or high-risk homebirth: An exploration of the literature on 'birthing outside the system'. *Midwifery*, 38, pp. 55–62.

Homer, C., Brodie, P., Sandall, J., and Leap, N. (2019). *Midwifery Continuity of Care: A Practical Guide*. London: Elsevier.

Jesse, D.E. and Reed, P.G. (2004). Effects of spirituality and psychosocial well-being on health risk behaviors in Appalachian pregnant women. *Journal of Obstetric, Gynecologic, Neonatal Nursing*, 33, pp. 739–747.

Kalmanofsky, A. (2008). Israel's baby: The horror of childbirth in the biblical prophets. *Biblical Interpretation*, 16, pp. 60–82.

Kay, L., Downe, S., Thomson, G., and Finlayson, K. (2017). Engaging with birth stories in pregnancy: A hermeneutic phenomenological study of women's experiences across two generations. *BMC Pregnancy and Childbirth*, 17, pp. 283–283.

Kildea, S. and Wardaguga, M. (2009). Childbirth in Australia: Aboriginal and Torress Strait Islander women. In: H. Selin and P.K. Stone eds, *Childbirth across Cultures: Ideas and Practices of Pregnancy, Childbirth and the Postpartum*. New York: Springer, pp. 275–286.

Kirkham, M. (2007). *Exploring the Dirty Side of Women's Health*. Oxon, UK: Routledge.

Kirkham, M. (2010). *The Midwife–Mother Relationship*. London: Palgrave Macmillan Limited.

Kitzinger, S. (2011). *Rediscovering Birth*. London: Pinter and Martin Ltd.

Kitzinger, S. (2012). Rediscovering the social model of childbirth. *Birth*, 39, pp. 301–304.

Lamaze, F. (1956). *Painless Childbirth: Psychoprophylactic Method*. Washington, D.C.: H. Regnery Co.

Leboyer, F. (1991). *Birth without Violence*. London: Mandarin.

Lewis, M., Jones, A., and Hunter, B. (2017). Women's experience of trust within the midwife–mother relationship. *International Journal of Childbirth*, 7, pp. 40–52.

Llewelyn Davis, M. (1915/1978). *Maternity: Letters from Working Women Collected by the Women's Co-operative Guild*. London: Virago.

Lokugamage, A. (2011). *The Heart in the Womb*. London: Docamali Limited.

Mander, R. (2004). *Men and Maternity*. London: Routledge.

McAra-Couper, J., Jones, M., and Smythe. L. (2012). Caesarean-section, my body, my choice: The construction of 'informed choice' in relation to intervention in childbirth. *Feminism & Psychology*, 22, pp. 81–97.

McIntosh, T. (2012). *A Social History of Maternity and Childbirth: Key Themes in Maternity Care*. London: Routledge.

Murphy-Lawless, J. (1998). *Reading Birth and Death*. Indianapolis, IN: Indiana University Press.

Murray, M. (2007). The magical female in Graeco-Roman Rabbinic literature. *Religion & Theology*, 14, pp. 284–309.

Myles, M. (1971). *Textbook for Midwives*. London: Churchhill Livingston.

Naraindas, H. (2009). A sacramental theory of childbirth in India. In: H. Selin and P.K. Stone eds, *Childbirth across Cultures: Ideas and Practices of Pregnancy, Childbirth and the Postpartum*. New York: Springer, pp. 95–105.

Odent, M. (2001). *The Scientification of Love*. London: Free Association Books.

Odent, M. (2002). *The Farmer and the Obstetrician*. London: Free Association Books Ltd.

Page, L. (1995). *Effective Group Practice in Midwifery: Working with Women*. Oxford, UK: Blackwell Science.

Pairman, S. (2010). Midwifery partnership: A professionalizing strategy for midwives. In: M. Kirkham, ed., *The Midwife–Mother Relationship*. London: Palgrave Macmillan Limited.

Riley, M. (1968). *Brought to Bed*. London: Dent and Sons Ltd.

Rimene, C., Hassan, C., and Broughton, J. (1998). *Ukaipo: The Place of Nurturing, Maori Women and Childbirth*. A Maori, Dunedin, NZ: Te Roopa Rangahau Hauora Maori o Ngai Tahu (the Ngai Tahu Maori health research unit), University of Otago.

Sandall, J., Soltani, H., Gates, S., Shennan, A., and Devane, D. (2016). Midwife-led continuity models versus other models of care for childbearing women. *Cochrane Database of Systematic Reviews*, 4, n.p.

Savage, W. (1986). *A Savage Enquiry: Who Controls Childbirth?* London: Virago.

Scamell, M. (2014). Childbirth within the risk society. *Sociology Compass*, 8, pp. 917–928.

Schneider, D.A. (2012). The miracle bearers: Narratives of birthing women and implications for spiritually informed social work practice. *Journal of Social Service Research*, 38, pp. 212–230.

Selin, H. and Stone, P.K. (2009). Childbirth across cultures: Ideas and practices of pregnancy, childbirth and the postpartum. *Science across Cultures: The History of Non-western Medicine*. New York: Springer.

Smith, J., Plaat, F., and Fisk, N.M. (2008). The natural caesarean: A woman-centred technique. *BJOG: An International Journal of Obstetrics and Gynaecology*, 115, pp. 1037–1041.

Smythe, E. (2010). Safety is an interpretive act: A hermeneutic analysis of care in childbirth. *International Journal of Nursing Studies*, 47, pp. 1474–1482.

Smythe, E., Hunter, M., Gunn, J., Crowther, S., Couper, J.M., Wilson, S., and Payne, D. (2016). Midwifing the notion of a 'good' birth: A philosophical analysis. *Midwifery*, 37, pp. 25–31.

Smythe, E., Payne, D., Wilson, S., *et al.* (2014). Providing a safe space for birth in Warkworth, New Zealand. In: R.C. White, ed., *Global Case Studies in Maternal and Child Health*. Burlington, MA: Jones & Bartlett Learning, pp. 187–208.

Stockham, A. (1890). *Tokology: A Book for Every Woman*. Chicago, IL: Alice Stockham and Co.

Stoll, K. and Hall, W.A. (2013). Attitudes and preferences of young women with low and high fear of childbirth. *Qualitative Health Research*, 23, pp. 1495–1505.

Stone, P.K. (2009). A history of western medicine, labor, and birth. In: H. Selin and P.K. Stone, eds, *Childbirth across Cultures: Ideas and Practices of Pregnancy, Childbirth and the Postpartum*. New York: Springer, pp. 41–53.

Styles, M. and Moccia, P. (1993). *On Nursing: A Literary Celebration*. New York: National League for Nursing Press.

Thackeray, W.M. and Pollard, A. (1847/1978). *Vanity Fair*. London: Macmillan.

Tong, R. (2009). *Feminist Thought: A More Comprehensive Introduction*. Boulder, CO: Westview Press.

Trevathan, W. (1987). *Human Birth: An Evolutionary Perspective*. New York: Aldine de Gruyter.

Ulrich, L.T. (1991). *A Midwife's Tale: The Life of Martha Ballard, Based on Her Diary 1785–1812*. New York: Vintage Books.

Walsh, L.V. (2009). Childbirth in the Mayan communities. In: H. Selin and P.K. Stone eds, *Childbirth across Cultures: Ideas and Practices of Pregnancy, Childbirth and the Postpartum*. New York: Springer, pp. 255–264.

Webb, J. and Fellowes, J. (2012). *Downton Abbey*. Series 3, Episode 5, ITV network, UK: Carnival Films.

Weir, L. (2006). *Pregnancy, Risk and Biopolitics: On the Threshold of the Living Subject*. New York: Routledge.

Worth, J. (2002). *Call the Midwife*. Twickenham, UK: Merton Books.

Yanagisawa, S. (2009). Childbirth in Japan. In: H. Selin and P.K. Stone eds, *Childbirth across Cultures: Ideas and Practices of Pregnancy, Childbirth and the Postpartum.* New York: Springer, pp. 85–94.

Zielinski, R., Ackerson, K., and Low, L.K. (2015). Planned home birth: Benefits, risks, and opportunities. *International Journal of Women's Health,* 7, p. 361.

Zisken, F.K. (2002). Dear God. *Judaism,* 51, p. 94.

Part II

A journey of poiesis

In the previous section you were invited into the beginning of a clearing through various horizons of understanding. The next four chapters present rich description and interpretation of the phenomenon joy at birth and invite you into a journey of poiesis.

In other research projects poiesis are often termed findings, however, in hermeneutic phenomenology the term 'findings' is misleading. The findings are in fact 'makings': a poiesis. Poiesis is from the Greek word 'ποίησις' to make. In this sense the Heideggerian interpretation is used implying a threshold moment (Heidegger, 2000). This moment is a process of bringing forth into appearance something from the experiential data of participant transcribed interviews that flowed from description and interpretation like the threshold of frozen river water melting in spring; a moment when the melted flowing water releases water from its frozenness un-concealing a plethora of remembered meanings. Poiesis is thus making something from the revelation of what was forgotten and concealed when one thing(s) becomes another. Poiesis is a horizon of interpretation that is on-the-way; it is thus a making not a finding.

This poiesis avoids readymade frameworks and allows the phenomenon of joy at birth to show itself unencumbered by previously fixed notions. To examine the whole of joy at birth could not be understood in isolation. Themes within the interpretive process slide and fold over each other, moving as they do from parts to whole and back in dialectical play. Remaining open to whatever possibilities are revealed allows a constant being-on-the-way of an unfolding 'poiesis' or 'makings'.

Reference

Heidegger, M. (2000). *Introduction to Metaphysics*. New Haven and London: Yale University Press.

Part II

A journey of poiesis

4 Making joy at birth visible

There is such a thing as joy at birth. This chapter both reveals its presence and claims that it is worthy of attention. The moment of joy is intangible and hidden within the lived-experience of being at birth. Heidegger draws attention to the invisibility of such moods and their evanescent and temporary quality. Furthermore, mood can be awoken or left sleeping until we turn towards it.

> Whatever is sleeping is in a peculiar way absent and yet there. When we awaken an attunement, this means that it is already there. At the same time, it expresses the fact that in a certain way it is not there. This is strange; attunement is something that is simultaneously there and not there.
>
> (Heidegger, 1995: 60)

The possibility of revealing something as elusive as a mood required a particular way of accessing. Through examining the emotions, feelings, and passions that arose in participant's stories, a background mood of joy at birth as common experience began to be uncovered, as Heidegger (1927/1962) suggests, "pointing something out is, by its very meaning, an uncovering" (271). For example, transient visible affective states or ontic moods provided a hint of what was sought. They gestured to an unseen and covered up mood at birth. Through the concretising of affective moods, distinctions were found that uncovered an onto-logical pre-reflective grounding attunement at birth embedded in complex con-texts. The themes illustrated in this chapter describe how birth attunement is made visible through the recognition of distinctions that danced and slid over one another bringing forth the first of the poiesis – *joy becomes un-concealed through disturbance of the taken-for-granted at birth.*

Safeguarding/sheltering at birth

Stories of sheltering and safeguarding something at birth reveal how participants knew *something* needed careful handling:

> It's unfortunate in a lot of ways that we have to open our packs, because they make noisy rustling and instruments too can make a bit of a noise if you're not careful I'm just trying to do it quietly and surreptitiously.... It's

like interjecting into something that is normal and natural with a sort of medical aspect. However, much I keep a birth normal, and aim for that, there are just always little things that I think are intrusive.

(Diane – midwife)

Diane, an experienced midwife, reveals a protective mode of activity and tries to create and safeguard a particular mood at birth. Even the rustle of opening delivery packs worries her because she is concerned that the mood at birth will be disrupted. She moves around the birth in ways that shelter and protects something precious. Shelter, in Heideggerian terms, is that which conceals harboured possibilities of our existence. To shelter something implies the hint of something, in this case a specific attuned mood at birth. The stories of sheltering hint at something mysterious that is safeguarded at birth. To safeguard is "to set something free into its own essence" (Heidegger, 1971/2001), in other words, to safeguard is an activity that strives for something to continue to be what it is. Diane's safeguarding *something* at birth provided the opportunity for this *something* to awaken and presence. What is the '*something*' that is safeguarded and sheltered? Can ways of being at birth *guard and shelter* joy so that it awakens?

Solicitous care[1]

Tui, a grandmother, tells a story of a rushed midwife and the sense of loss of something she felt from this midwife's solicitous care:

> It was a strange birth; it wasn't long but the midwife, when my daughter didn't want to push, just reached in and pulled the baby. It was a strange feeling for me, it felt the time had been rushed. I knew that everything was alright. I didn't have any doubts. But when baby arrived, when I saw the head, it felt too fast. It was rushed because of the midwife's actions. That is the only birth that I haven't felt that real joy. We had to quickly adjust as it was a jolt, we weren't ready for it. My daughter quickly adjusted because she had to. For me, it was a bit harder. I held my granddaughter afterwards, but it wasn't nice. It was lovely to see this beautiful baby being born, but it wasn't that same feeling, it didn't flow.

(Tui)

This midwife, according to Tui, did not know how to get her mode of care right. Her rushed actions altered the mood of joy at this birth. This story is one of disappointment, the flow of events disrupted due to the midwife's way of caring. Tui is upset by the seemingly rushed way the midwife 'leaped-in' and took control, speeding things along. She tries to reconcile her feeling by acknowledging that her daughter was distraught and needed assistance but despite this felt that something was disrupted and taken from her. The birth felt like 'a jolt' that they 'were not ready for'. Tui was left feeling that it could have been handled differently. The joy at her granddaughter's birth was not honoured.

Mother and baby were well, but something was lacking, and Tui felt bereft and deprived of the joy at birth that she had come to expect.

Solicitous care is guarding and sheltering something at birth. Something of the nature of an ungraspable mood at birth is revealed in the solicitous modes of leaping-in and leaping-ahead as sheltering and guarding. Yet these are not mutually exclusive modes of being; one is not necessarily better than another. Neither are participants always going to get the optimal mode of solicitous care right or achieve it. As Joshua Spiers (2019) further illustrates care cannot be placed in clearly defined categories of leaping-in and leaping-ahead so easily. They are situation dependent. Leaping-in care could be the best care on occasions so that someone can leap-ahead into their own unfolding future possibilities. The tension is always to know when to do what. It's the wisdom, tact or perhaps indeterminate ways of being that helps get that right, known by mood.

The feeling of being invaded physically and left bereft of joy at birth is highlighted in several stories when care does not shelter or safeguard the mood at birth:

> It was interesting, when there were people in the room, it felt more stressful. I remember another midwife or another nurse wanting to watch, asking Dina [Cathy's midwife] if she could watch what she was doing because she wanted to see how she did it and wanted to learn from it. There was just a lot more busyness. It was more stressful; I was less calm when there were more people in the room. I think it's because they're all working towards you and working on you but not working with you. Once everyone left it was easier to calm down. The lights were dimmed again. The mood changed and I could rest more. It was a restful calm mood as opposed to the busy hospital room.
>
> (Cathy – mother)

The behaviour of hospital staff alienated Cathy. They were '*working towards you and working on you but not working with you*'. Her description is not so much critical but an observation of the calming influence and positive difference once they left. Exposing solicitous care (leaping-in and leaping-ahead) draws further attention to a specific mood at birth that can be sheltered or disrupted, made absent or present by how others enact care.

Protecting 'something' at birth

Pat talks of surrendering to something special at birth. Leaping-in with interventions for Pat would be the anathema to her wishes. The mood at birth was important and needed to be protected. She explains why:

> It's definitely a time to surrender, we needed to surrender and accept that Mother Nature, God or whoever has got it all under control. That mood of surrender is quite powerful, having faith and trust in that it is all going to go the way it needs to go. The result will be the result we require to help us on to the next stage of our lives.
>
> (Pat)

Pat speaks of a knowing, faith, trust, and ultimate surrender to the powerful forces at play in the process of birthing that she experienced. Her belief system is pivotal to her understanding birth; she is attuned to birth in a certain way. The birth would play out in accordance to some preordained divine process that needs protecting and sheltering. For Pat, the meaning of birth is connected with surrendering to this natural process. She speaks of being a conduit for life to express itself through her. This story reveals something significant at birth and a mood at birth that requires others to leap-ahead in their solicitude allowing sheltered possibilities to surface. She cares about attuning joyfully at birth as this, she believes, is something precious and beneficial to the process. Participant midwives also care about preserving something precious at birth:

> I want to respect the sacred thing that's happening, and I don't want to impede it. I think you can impede it by invoking the rationality of things by engaging rationally with women when they should be doing what their body tells them to do; so that they can access the instinctive stuff. Like this woman yesterday she needed the time, but the obstetrician wanted me to break her waters for high blood pressure. I tried to create the space for her to do what she [birthing woman] needed to do.
>
> (Simone – midwife)

Simone describes her frustration at how others, in this case the obstetrician, can disrupt and disturb the mood at birth that she treasures. This mood in this story appears vulnerable to the intrusive nature of rushing into doing things. The obstetrician appears to be leaping-in, interfering, and disrupting the ability of this mother to cope with labour and birth. Simone is demonstrating leaping-ahead and avoids hasty interventions. She accuses the obstetrician of lacking the sensitivity to see how labour reveals itself. She thinks that such leaping-in unnecessarily dominates and takes over birth and relates to the obstetrician's need to control the process and, in doing so, impedes something of importance at birth. As Heidegger suggests "… that which leaps in…dominates, and that which leaps forth … liberates" (Heidegger, 1927/1962: 159). Simone's care was focused on a desire to liberate so that something special at birth could arrive.

These stories highlight the way caring influences the lived-experience of mood at birth. Being-in-the-world-of-birth is one of care indicating how all are enmeshed in the world of birth experiences. Mood at birth, here named joy, reveals itself more in the way participants care about birth and the nature of solicitude. It is through such care that the mood at birth is revealed as significant. Care implies significance, something of worth, and a relational interconnected totality of the whole birth experience. The need to be at birth in a particular way and attune in certain ways uncovers how birth matters to participants.

Dwelling at birth in a particular way

There is a sense of how participants desire to dwell within something at birth. For Heidegger (1971/2001) to dwell is to spare and preserve a place where we are at peace. Throughout many of the stories the centrality of calmness is revealed. Calmness, in its different descriptions, is often juxtaposed with instances of disturbance and interference. It appears that attuning to calmness is a notion significant to birth. Some participants reported feeling anguish when the calmness of birth was broken:

> There was this amazement that all this was happening so quietly; it was the first birth I was at. I was just amazed about the process. The silence keeps coming back to me. It's probably why now when I hear women screaming, I have an internal reaction because there was something of the quietness of birth that amazed me.
>
> (Marie – midwife)

This story of Marie's first birth experience speaks of innocence, wonder, and amazement. But it is the silence and quietness of the birth that strikes her and revisits her daily in her work as a midwife 40 years later. Yet how is it possible to think or speak of silence? Silence is "…almost by its nature, is unspeakable…" (Rethmann, 2006: 44). The silence keeps coming back to Marie as something essentially part of this miraculous process. She remembers lucidly the sense of silence and quietness. She is surprised by the simplicity juxtaposed to the miracle unfolding right there in the room in front of her surrounded by calmness and silence. She continues:

> I get thrown when something happens like this instrumental birth. It's not a failure on anybody's part, violence is too strong a word, but when you have had a quiet, gentle, respectful intimate thing like yesterday, then suddenly (raises her voice and opens arms) THE LIGHTS ARE ON, EXTRA PEOPLE ARE THERE AND ITS ALL A HISS AND ROAR. That is why I still have difficulty about being rational afterwards. I don't think I have failed but it is the opposite of the gentle physiological birth. An intimate thing changed into something else. After all these years I can look at it and say that it is okay when the outcome was good, yet I don't feel that it is always okay.
>
> (Marie – midwife)

Marie's story illustrates how the calmness is disturbed and how she is literally 'thrown'. It is in stories of disturbance that a special mood at birth is revealed. When the gentle quietness at birth is shattered, Marie finds herself suddenly attuned to anguish. Once disturbed, it is difficult to regain the intimate nature of birth. She continues:

> It is just that prayer and reflection is important in my life and I know that stillness is a huge part of letting go. For me it is about letting the process happen and being ready to intervene if it does not.
>
> (Marie)

Stillness is important for Marie. In her own life and spiritual belief systems she sees stillness and calmness as a way of facilitating the letting go. She finds it difficult to reconcile when birth is disturbed. The dramatic changes in the physical environment move from a gentle intimate calmness into something public and disturbing. The quest for silence is echoed in many other participant stories and I am reminded in my own practice of how childbirth can be thrown into a dance between the frantic features of emergencies whilst remaining sympathetic to the calmness of birth. There seems to be something fundamental and basic in the desire to shelter calm at births.

Jennifer De Leon's study about dance (2005) uncovered how stillness is healing and transformative. She found that within chaos and activity a moment of stillness can be transformed into wisdom in which a sense of connection with oneself and with others is engendered:

> ... a transpersonal sense of Something greater and beyond the dance ... an ecstatic sense of aliveness imparting the ability to transcend fixedness and supporting the capability to maintain integrity and a sense of self in the midst of turmoil ... [an] engagement and connectedness with presence.
>
> (103)

Marie dwells in a particular way at birth that gives her freedom to shelter, preserve, and guard that special peaceful quality at birth even within turmoil. It appears that attuning to the stillness and silence of birth provides an opportunity for the authentic to surface and be known. Marie's experiences thus reveal a mood specific to birth that she prefers to dwell within. This dwelling is akin to remaining home at birth for Marie. Heidegger (1971/2001) argues that many of us have forgotten how to truly dwell whilst in the speed of modern life, although we are never completely severed from home, we are at the same time never completely at home.

For Marie disturbance in stillness and calm at birth is challenging to reconcile. To dwell in a place of stillness at birth, even in times of childbirth intervention, perhaps awakens the possibility to attune '*in the right way*' transforming anxiety to joyful calm. Midwife participants spoke of feeling unsettled at how the beauty of quietness at birth is disrupted by others who appear to lack sensitivity to the mood. Anahera [Māori midwife] expresses her concerns about noise and how disrupting calm can cover up '*something*' at birth:

> We were all calm. I don't like people coming in and being loud and getting stressed. I don't like midwives walking in disturbing. If I call them in, I don't make a big scene about it. I like babies to come into their world calmly with a controlled mother. If mothers start screaming, I let them have their moment of screaming, and then I'll pull them back in. That's part of my job to bring them back to themselves. A calm birthing room is about everyone being in that state of mind, in that feeling that goes nicely with meeting the baby. We're all excited about meeting the baby; for most families it's a really joyous time. But I feel like that moment of joy can be

overridden by fear and chaos. I go into some rooms where birthing women are screaming down the house and it just sounds like a room of fear. I just think for our little ones that have to hear that when they're being born, I find that incredibly sad, but obviously that is their little journey.

Importance of dwelling in calmness at birth is highlighted by Anehera. The main aspect of Anahera's midwifery practice, other than facilitating safety, is to facilitate a favourable mood into which the baby is born. She reveals how joy at birth can be obscured by chaos, noise, and franticness leaving birth fearfully attuned. Midwife participants frequently hinted at something of significance being absent at births during noisy frantic disruptions. They treasure the calmness that greets a baby and have a sense of responsibility for holding and protecting this essential part of birth.

An essential attunement (mood) at birth

It appears that an essential attunement can remain sleeping in times of disruption. I am reminded of midwives guarding the mood of birth in other stories and not letting it dissipate or "guarding against it falling asleep" (Heidegger, 1995: 79). In a seeming paradox, the noisy chaotic birth acts soporifically to the mood at birth that midwives attempt to shelter. The way midwife participants practice gestures something in the silence and stillness that often remains unnamed. Their concerning practices point to the presence of a special mood at birth that needs sheltering and safeguarding. They reported feeling honoured to be part of this journey, taking on their role at birth seriously and attuning with reverence and sensitivity.

Whatever the rationale for midwives' actions, mothers too speak of their need for calm as labour flows into birth:

There was this need to be in a real still silent space. By silent I guess I mean "Still" – no mind chatter. It was one of the few times in my life that I genuinely did not have to deal with any mind chatter and felt really focused and happy.

(Amy – mother)

Amy speaks of the importance of silence and stillness. The inward focus facilitated by the stillness reduces the internal voices so that she is able to turn towards and awaken the joy at birth. The breaking of this stillness and calmness through unwarranted leaping-in modes of care appears to disrupt this turning towards and awakening of joy at birth. The stillness and calmness at birth seems important to the process and deeply meaningful. There is the announcement of joy as Amy describes this stillness and its meaning at the birth of her baby:

There was a great sense of hope and optimism. There was this great sense of divinity, a kind of stillness. There is a great sense of joy at that moment.

The safe arrival of a baby enriches the lived-experiences in expected ways. The power of joy at birth is evident. Amy attunes to hope and optimism that gesture to future yet-to-be-realised possibilities. However, it is a 'great' joy that brings the experience into wholeness. This joy at birth is beautifully expressed by Amy when her baby is delivered in the unexpected turmoil of a forceps delivery. Despite the mode of birth, joy awakens from stillness hinting at something divine in nature that fills Amy with hope and optimism.

A quality of calmness at birth is revealed as constitutive of the experience. Yet this calmness can be disrupted and beckons and yearns to be sheltered and safeguarded. Participants show how they care about mood at birth becoming custodians of something so that it continues to 'be'. By safeguarding 'it' they ensure its continuance holding it safe from harm. In their sheltering and safeguarding practices, they remain available to joy's arrival.

Joy's arrival

Another quality of joy at birth is 'suddenness'. Something powerful and over-whelming arrives at birth that those there find themselves bursting into tears:

> At the C. Section there are the bright lights, a lot of people, and if it's an emergency situation there is all this uncertainty. This is fear for the Mum's and baby's well-being. When that baby is born because of the situation it is out and handed to paediatricians. Sometimes the obstetrician will lower the curtain and show the baby. Then there is this void time of waiting. The elation isn't there immediately but from seeing the baby comes the joy. When the baby is finally given to the mother then tears of joy, the welcoming, touching and quiet voices and meeting of the family. It happens afterwards; after a 5 to 10 minutes time lag.
>
> (Selene – midwife)

In situations of intervention it seems the joy at birth either irrupts instantly or after a delay, but still with a sense of suddenness. From nowhere and every-where joy floods into the room revealing the occasion as special and significant. Participants reveal joy as delayed due to intervention and more specifically because of lack of contact with the parents. Selene describes a situation in which the mother is under general anaesthetic:

> There was this crash section three weeks ago under GA.[2] The mother is unconscious and so Dad was out of the theatre. For me the joy was being there to welcome this baby, I spoke to the baby, touched the baby and wrapped the baby in warm towels and held the baby. Then the second midwife took the baby to Dad straightaway, skin to skin. I felt absolutely relieved when I saw the baby being lifted out as it had been really traumatic crash run to theatre. I was overcome completely with relief because it had been a situation where there was serious brachycardia;[3] it was one of those life-death situations. When I heard the baby cry, I just smiled because everything is good and right. This baby's fine and there's the joy, it was there. However, it is not quite the same until the parents experience their baby; that's really when I feel that explosion of joy.
>
> (Simone – midwife)

There is relief following the anxious events leading to the delivery. This sense of relief once the physical aspects are completed is a common theme throughout participant narratives. When it is apparent the baby is well, joy arrives as if waiting for the right moment. There is an irrupting joy as the parents first meet their baby after delay. What is significant is that there is joy at birth despite the milieu of intervention. Paradoxically the need for life saving intervention acts to hold hope of a yet-to-awaken joy even if that joy must be delayed. The leaping in enables the leaping ahead into possibilities. The baby's safe arrival and first meeting with the parents enriches the lived-experience in those precious initial moments in palpable and expected ways. In an instant they become free to discover the possibilities of a new life together.

For *something* to arrive suddenly, even after delay, implies that it already and always exists. For joy to be waiting or absent means that it is merely away, on its way, soon to arrive; not non-existent. Brenda, a junior obstetrician, illuminates this further and tells of how joy is always there despite medical intervention and describes how joy eventually arrives:

> We had a lady with twins in premature labour at 28 weeks. The decision was to do a caesarean as the first twin was breech. The whole family is there and it's very tense, all are scared. The paediatricians had come to talk to them about potential outcomes and prognosis. The first baby came out fine. Then the second baby was delivered in its gestational sack. The consultant slowly eased this little sack out, you could see this little baby still swimming around with its hair floating like a little mermaid; its hands bouncing against the sack. It was so slow and controlled and then she popped the sack in which this little thing was. The baby splattered out and started breathing. The Dad looked over and instantly on seeing his baby burst into tears. Then the mother burst into tears. Tears of relief and joy ... [Pause and smiling] of amazement. I was focused on the medical right up until I could see the safe delivery. That moment is present in every birth but there's just some in which it's stronger. I think at this one it was very strong.
>
> (Brenda – obstetrician)

The mood of fear and tenseness that is seemingly a part of Brenda's work is evident. Yet the joy awakens eventually bringing into relief its existence. The stress is palpable in stories in which obstetricians are called to assist. Everyone is tense until the babies are delivered by caesarean section. Yet something magical occurs in the birth of the second baby as Brenda can peer into another world. Within the same high-risk experience as if deeply asleep until awakened, joy assails suddenly after delay.

There is a mysterious otherworldly quality in Brenda's story. The consultant she assists is slow and controlled and eases the fragile tiny twin into the world. Then there is an outpouring of emotion following a delay in response to the changed mood initiated by relief. A unifying joy floods into the room that is so powerful and overwhelming that the father and mother burst into tears. There is a timeless quality to the attunement that is, as Heidegger (1995) reminds us, "Neither merely the present not merely the past nor merely the future, nor indeed all these reckoned together" (148). There is something about joy that completes and makes whole something extraordinary at birth. Even in times of adversity when anxiety and the potential for sorrow are awakened, they give way to the awakening of joy. Brenda says that it is a medical act up to that moment but something powerful shifts at birth. Joy at birth shows itself as having a totalising and gathering power despite being delayed.

However, those at birth appear vulnerable to influences that can turn them away and force them out from this moment of joy. Being forced from one mood into another also reveals more of the quality of suddenness. Amy [mother] speaks of her forceps birth and relates how she felt suddenly jolted out of being joyfully attuned:

> I was not feeling joy. There was a big sense of feeling degraded in these stirrups, just that position in itself felt very disempowering. I was okay up until the lights got turned on full and the obstetrician came in. She was a bit cold and not very communicative. The legs went in stirrups [clicks her fingers] and there was a lot that changed very quickly; all of a sudden there was this team of people who came into the room … doing things around me. My midwife tried to prepare me for that, but it was the obstetrician what changed everything. I can remember when Ellie was crowning, and the forceps are there. The obstetrician pretty much just guided her head out. I did most of the force myself. The obstetrician had the awareness to say that to me, but her hands felt really foreign, she hurt more than anybody else. She was a very good mechanic, she did her job very well, but she wasn't totally connected to me or the situation. Her approach did snap that sacred space out. I think that it's a fundamental basis for me, being in that sacred space.
>
> (Amy)

Amy felt violated by the suddenness of the events unfolding. It was as if she was forcibly pulled from joy to despair. She refers to this as being snapped out of sacred space. The unexpected vulnerability and suddenness of her thrownness means that the experience becomes unenjoyable. The obstetrician is efficient at what she does but remains disconnected. The lights are turned on without consent and a different mood floods the room. Anxiety is awakened; fear replaces joy as a medicalised hospital event unfolds. The previous mood, which she names as sacred, is covered over by an avalanche of other feelings which undermine the prior sacred and joy. The voices of the One penetrate into the private and intimate space. The intimate atmosphere is broken. The occasion is now one of hospital routines and unknown others.

As with other similar stories when lights are put on it seems everyone is forced out of the proceeding calmness and stillness. Switching on lights is analogous with flooding the room with a different mood that awakens anxiety and fear. In this abrupt disturbance a backgrounded mood at birth is further revealed as joy's sudden withdrawal into absence reveals once more how joy becomes startlingly known in its 'not there' presence. Paradoxically joy at birth becomes visibly absent.

Mothers, birth partners, and midwives try desperately to maintain a modicum of joy at birth in the context of medicalised hospital events that seek to shelter physical safety of mother and baby. Perhaps there is something quintessentially embodied in the desire to protect calmness at births; a sense of safeguarding something sacred, of holding, and protecting a precious gift. I am reminded how the sudden 'jolt' from one mood to another can leave something at birth in darkness. The sudden arrival of mood is akin to the way Heidegger describes how moods quickly overcome us: "[taking] hold ... in an instant like a flash of lightening" (Heidegger, 1995: 148).

The fact that moods can be changed attests to their presence as we are always attuned somehow in every situation. To feel joy's absence and yearn for its arrival is to honour that it exists. Participants have described the possibility to turn towards joy and turn away from fear that reveals their experiences at birth in different ways. This would seem significant and beckons questions: 'Can those at birth influence and awaken joy at birth?' and 'If joy is not attuned to at birth what can be done to awaken it?'

Childbirth technology and joy

Joy at birth is significant and meaningful but can be delayed and hidden by disturbances and interference pointing to how different ways of care in maternity practice can guard and shelter or disturb. The technocratic infrastructure now ubiquitous in western twenty-first century maternity wards and systems does not necessarily conceal or prevent joy at birth because joy at birth becomes visible in myriad unexpected circumstances:

> The vulnerability of being with legs tied up, forceps and pain, it was dreadful. However, I still don't have any regrets. It felt like a real journey for me and there was something very necessary about every part of it. There was gold in every part of it even the dreadful last bit. It was dreadful, but it wasn't. It was what was needed. I remember feeling very teary very quickly when she was out. Like an intense wave of emotion. I had an immediate sense of empowerment that came back. The emotion was love. It was a pretty whole-body experience I think of love and reverence. It was just this feeling of reverence and I'm like "Wow", it's happened, a wow moment. The reverence was just like having all your hands up like that [hands rose] to be a witness to the wonder. Witnessing and experiencing that spark of preciousness and to see it in that moment. Reverence − it can mean lots of things, but I think that's what it means.
>
> (Amy – mother)

Amy speaks of a reconciling of the emotional turmoil that Ellie's birth brings. She speaks of the dreadfulness of the forceps experience but then tells of how she incorporates this aspect of her daughter's birth in a greater whole. She spontaneously brings meaning to this part by looking at the whole of her childbirth experience. For Amy, this was a journey of self-discovery, a voyage into motherhood. Each part of the journey, she reflects, is a bit of gold. The significance of the whole and not the parts in isolation are again highlighted.

Even amidst the dreadfulness she relates the awesome wholeness of the first encounter, the sense of awe, wonder, gratitude, and reverence. She describes a love at birth which captivates and overcomes her describing this as a 'spark of preciousness'. Like an alchemic process, the second stage of labour and the moments after birth reveal gold from the dark places that went before. The mix of powerful feelings as the birth unfolded transforms the occasion despite the technocratic positioning of the birth experience. Amy's birth appears to be made of many elements that provide a rich layered story of joyous attunement at birth. The tensions in her story further revealed the power and potency of joy at birth.

The magnitude of interference in Amy's story is incorporated and fused with wonder revealing an essential paradox. Being positioned within childbirth technology has saved her baby from harm and enriched her journey to motherhood. If her baby had come to harm, joy would have retreated into shadow as she became attuned instead to sorrow.

Joy and sorrow have been understood as co-existing in experience because either one can surface depending on the situation (Parse, 1997). Anxiety and joy as attuning possibilities are always available in experience yet when joy arrives it is fully realised and complete when not accompanied by anxiety (Smith, 1981). What is significant is that joy at birth can surface when things go well, revealing an awakened presence of joy through the milieu of technology. Equally there is a possibility of attuning anxiously as challenging medical events unfold and an awakening sorrow if things end badly. There is a sense that joy is intensified due to this co-existence within a continual possibility of anxiety and sorrow. The awakening of joy at birth has shown itself as relief in stories of high acuity and increased medical intervention. Joy through disturbance and challenges becomes visible.

Westernised childbirth is now positioned within technology informing the thinking and discourse around birth. Positionality[4] is a term coined by Heidegger that sees technology as ordered revealing, gathering, and restructuring that constantly closes possibilities of further revealing (Heidegger, 1993/1954). The privileging of technology over natural approaches often provokes polemic debates as discussed in Chapter 2. Yet from this phenomenological inquiry focused on 'joy at birth' has found that birthing technology is not wanting; positive or negative. What is evident is that technology can shelter and protect that which is precious, maintaining the possibility for joy to awaken even when delayed as in high risk births. Even in high interventionist births, participants speak of joy and elation.

Birth technology can close possibilities but equally holds the potential to provide opportunity to attune joyfully at birth when such joy would not have arrived. However, concerns that technology and modern maternity care disturb, prevent and hide a joyful birth need further questioning. Heidegger (1993/1954) might argue that opening ourselves to the essence of birthing technology would free us in our projects. I am cognisant of this Heideggerian orientation but also acknowledge that technology and the bio-medical approach to birth can pose tension as apparent different worlds meet and/or collide. This perceptible tension provides further glimpses of joy at birth that I seek to make visible and bring to language. As one thing collides with another something that was not seen or heard before surfaces. In that meeting of seeming opposites joy at birth calls out and is further revealed.

Although there are areas of conflict in western childbirth, it is evident from participant stories that they all care about birth from differing perspectives. Birth matters to them all. I would argue that their care, however that is enacted, gestures towards birth as meaningful. In addition to their concerns about safety, they care about how birth is attuned. This reveals the significance of joy at birth and highlights how birth matters in their modes of solicitous caring. Participants appeared to attune reverently and sensitively at birth, feeling frustrated when others disrupted and disturbed joy at birth. The vulnerable treasured joy that participants sought to protect is an essential part of their lived-experience at birth which matters to them.

> It was not about loss of control and power as I knew the baby needed to come out and needed help to do so, but it was that what had been a quiet respective thing suddenly became the opposite. I was relieved as one part of me knew we needed to get help. But I also felt disappointment for her as they had wanted this lovely normal private birth. There was certainly no fear in the atmosphere before. When I say the word violation it was the change in atmosphere, something special changed when the doctors came in, the lights were on, three unknown men entered, her legs were suddenly up in lithotomy, there was an unknown paediatrician, an extra midwife, lots of noise, the gentleness of it had been taken away, the silence was gone.
>
> (Marie – midwife)

Marie is deeply troubled. She highlights the disturbance due to different worlds colliding and meeting, revealing the cultural differences in the two main health care professionals involved at births; midwives and obstetricians. It was important that the baby and mother are well, and the parents are delighted to have a healthy baby in their arms, but Marie is haunted by the fact that silence had been replaced by anxiety, noise, and frantic activity. She accepts the fact the baby needed assistance to be born but is concerned about the way it was instigated without reverence or courtesy. The suddenness of medical intervention is construed negatively, and Marie laments the thrownness of such disrupted occasions. She continues:

> I could have understood it if it had been urgent; but it was not urgent. It was upsetting due to the lack of courtesy to the woman; I just couldn't believe that it was like that. In fact, I have not gone and spoken to them about it as it makes no difference and they will not listen anyway. I was mortified; I felt that I had betrayed her somehow, because I had not prepared her for that. I had gone for help but didn't know he was going to bring two others in and then spend another 5–10 minutes teaching the house surgeon how to put the cap on. I am

trying to be professionally collegial and not saying anything nasty to him, trying to be in partnership with the couple. I moved the student away to do the notes as I was trying to protect her from feeling upset and from this feeling that the atmosphere had changed suddenly. I wanted to protect her from being yelled at by an obstetrician, for not moving fast enough or handing him the wrong thing, as that had already happened to her by another obstetrician. Something changed in the atmosphere that made me feel different.

Marie encourages the process to be calm and quiet in order to turn towards and awaken joy at birth. The breaking of this stillness and handing over of the process to others creates a collision of perspectives experienced as a violent confrontational meeting that she attempts to shield the student from. Yet there are many perspectives and Carol [senior obstetrician] gives another:

I think most times the atmosphere in the room has already started to change before I get there; the tension level might have already risen. I know the patient and the family knows that the midwife has called the consultant and there's concern, there's some issues, maybe if it's a woman who's exhausted or in pain, she is already anxious. There's always a little bit of anxiety that's already started simply because the doctors had to be called. Something's going on. Sometimes I find that hard to be in that role; the one who's going to have to sort it out. I don't feel antagonism at all, it's not like I'm walking into a death trap or anything! Sometimes it is hard especially people who wanted everything without intervention and at home naturally and that's frustrating for people too.

Carol suggests that mood at birth is altered before she gets there because events are not going well. It is in these situations that she is called upon; that is her function in the maternity team – to attend when things are going wrong. There is usually associated stress and anxiety due to the nature of her being called in to help. Carol finds it difficult, professionally and personally, to come in and change plans and management of care that are not what the woman and family had originally hoped for. Carol is called upon to leap-in and help. The call of the doctor seems to be the harbinger of intervention and others' need for surrender to institutional processes rather than a calm joyous attuning.

However, something is revealed in this apparent tension. Something is altered in the doctor's arrival. The 'how' of Carol's obstetric actions reveals more of the joy at birth. She is aware of the potential impact of her ways of solicitous care on others. The meeting of different professional groups and family cultures reveals tensions in the lived-experiences at birth. Carol is similarly respectful and sensitive of others at birth whilst acknowledging the existence of joy at birth. She is certainly not divorced from joy at birth. She is aware of anxiety, the potential for sorrow, and her impact on others at birth and reflects further on this:

I'm a little surprised at how clinical I'm sounding and how lacking emotion I am! I realise that my job is different here than what I came from where I was more involved in the whole pregnancy of someone, versus here where I'm mostly involved with whatever issues it is at that moment. So, I'm much less emotionally involved here. Being emotionally connected allows me to get into that feeling of happiness more. You know that my job isn't necessarily to be happy at the birth, it's nice, I can feel nice when that's the case like a happy baby born into a lovely family, and it's a nice feeling. I think there's so much anticipation around the mother and her family and her partner having a baby; the baby is going to be their baby to love and raise and nurture and in our society that's a treasured thing to be able to do. So, in most cases it's a happy much anticipated event. It's something people have been longing for and looking forward to and therefore I'm happy when it's all going fine.

Carol narrates a sense of grief as she turns away from joyousness at birth inferring that joy exists. It is not her '*job to be happy at the birth*'. This reflection shows how Carol is denied the full experience of being immersed in a joyous mood. She turns away from the joy and thus paradoxically acknowledges it is present at birth. She is glad when all goes well but does not allow herself to fully experience joy's arrival. To be able to turn towards or away yet again reveals joy at birth. There is a sense of sadness as the wholeness of the birth experience for Carol becomes privative in some way. Carol's role as an obstetrician seemingly denies access to aspects of human experience at birth.

The convergence of differing professional and personal ways of being highlights the tensions within these experiences. Carol's primary concern is risk management and sorting things out when she is called. Despite the distinctions between medicine and midwifery, both traditions reveal the presence of joy at birth. It is plausible that birth holds special meaning to all natal beings, whoever and whatever roles they play in Being-in-the-world-of-birth. Carol expresses something about the universal power of joy at the following Ventouse birth:[5]

When this baby was out there was that happiness in the room. I would say it's pretty universal. I mean there might be some underlying emotions again about why the vacuum had to happen. What was going on? But I think overall, it's a universal happiness as there's now a baby in the room. I think there is happiness, a relief that finally this part is completed, and we have this end product. I think probably there is some sort of emotional thing there because otherwise we would neglect our babies and not feed them. It's one of those life events that have a lot of emotion tied to it. In that sense its special, but I don't think of birth as an epiphany or spiritual sacred event or anything like that, it's a part of life; it's a very normal life process that is special, that's all. It is not cosmic to me or spiritual or things like that. It's a normal part of life but one we attribute a lot of specialness too! There is something special going on; though I can't define special.

Carol struggles to find words to express how she experiences the joy at birth; yet she acknowledges the specialness of birth. The way Carol and other participants articulate their experiences is influenced by their pre-understandings, fore-structures, and effective histories (see previous chapter). The languaging – or way we name in words – 'joy at birth' differs but the sense of specialness is evident.

The history of conflict and difference amongst maternity care providers and service users as explored in Chapter 3 does not belong to the participants in this study. These conflicts belong to maternity care traditions of which they are part. The distinctions provided by these differences and challenges highlight joy at birth further. Joy at birth seemingly dances within and around these histories representing a coming together of differing understandings. I sought the differing perspectives conscientiously, eager not to privilege the voices of one group over another, albeit recognising the embodied nature of my own midwifery perspective. I sought common understanding through dialogue with these differences which uncovered more than was possible from singular individual perspectives.

Gadamer's (1960/1975) fusion of horizons shows how interpretations and understandings of events reveal what matters most at the heart of participant's actions in the world of birth. For example, it is only possible for Marie to interpret within her own culture of midwifery and for Carol to interpret within her medical tradition; perhaps neither fully appreciating the culture of the other. The midwifery profession and medical profession each has its own culture within which myriad interpretations and divisions have developed. For Marie, the silence and intimacy are central to birth and are entwined in the parent's wishes and expectations. For Carol, obstetric practices at birth are imbued with responsibility and risk reduction rather than being happy. Birth for Marie is a normal event unfolding in quiet gentle calmness that opens the birth experience to something more than a healthy birth outcome. Carol believes it is her responsibility to address problems.

Both obstetricians and midwives care about birth. It would seem a truism that birth is significant, yet they care about it in different ways. It can be inferred that this care arises due to the significance of birth that lies in the commonality of their worlds. For example, the sense of sacred or special articulated by Carol and Marie points to a commonality in their lived-experience. The history of their perspectives is not so much of worlds colliding, but of meeting and working together from different points of view. All participants in this inquiry belong to a western maternity care tradition constituted of different cultural points of view that make up that world.

Obstetricians practice within the world of medicine and acute hospital labour ward concerns. There is an interwoven totality of concerns that makes up their world. Obstetricians are often thrown into situations of high acuity at birth, situations they need to 'sort out', situations about which they are professionally concerned. This is particularly intense for obstetricians who represent the final frontier of those who can avert tragedy. The obstetric mood at birth is one of anxiety arising from responsibility in times of high acuity, risk, uncertainty, and unknown outcomes.

Conversely, midwives describe ways of guarding and sheltering at birth that is concerned with keeping awake and holding an attunement at birth that they treasure and understand as precious. Obstetricians have spoken about the specialness of birth and recognise the significance of the occasion juxtaposed to the notion of turning away from this mood of joy to do the medical job required of them. What is revealed in these differences is that birth is disclosed as significant through the arrival of joy at birth despite cultural differences. The existence of the phenomenon "Joy at birth" is made visible through these differences and is announced through different modes of solicitous care which in turn makes joy more visible.

Conclusion

This chapter has established that the phenomenon joy at birth exists, both in its presence and absence. Participant stories contain details of disruptions and distinctions. These reveal that 'something' almost intangible is inherent in the world of birth. They draw attention to what is experienced in addition to and beyond the average everyday experiences at birth. They assist us to see the 'something' at birth that is or is not there in the everyday taken-for-granted modern maternity care when all is going smoothly. Stories that sought to shelter, defend, and protect joy at birth from the disturbances and challenges brought the mood of joy at birth further into focus. Joy at birth is paradoxically a failure to see the attunement itself because it is always in the background just beyond our grasp. Yet, when joy at birth arrives suddenly, it is a shared experience which appears to sweep those present with an overwhelming intensity. We have also seen how the potential for sorrow and anxiety at birth recedes as joy awakens 'in a flash'. Joy can be awakened or left asleep, but it is always already there in lived-experience of birth. Moreover, joy at birth is so familiar and much a part of an everyday taken-for-granted experience at birth that it is rarely spoken about and perhaps at times ignored, lost, and forgotten. The power and gift of joy at birth is in the possibility it brings to eradicate, or lesson unpleasant feelings associated with any disruption or interference. The purpose of this chapter was to make visible the phenomenon 'joy at birth'. The key message is that joy at birth does exist hinting at profound and concealed meanings awaiting further un-concealment.

Sophia

Silence finds its way into the theatre today
wisdom fills the air –
The mystery unfolds
as Joy born again
This time,
into air through this mother's abdomen
I cry … you cry … we cry … our cry
green sheets, red blood and lots and lots and lots of things and doing!
Chaos abounds
technology gathers and saves
Yet Sophia, my silent love, you remain present
calling and radiating
a melodious blissful wonder

(Poem taken from my reflective diary – Sophia[6])

Notes

1 Solicitous care according to Heidegger is an activity or mode of caring of others who need help. There are two modes of solicitude: Leaping-in, a taking over of the other's project, a mode of care that dominates the other that can lead to dependency and leaping-ahead that is concerned with allowing others to carry out their own projects and become more transparent to themselves in their coping.
2 Crash caesarean section denotes an emergency and need for unplanned surgery to save either or both the woman and infant from harm. GA – means a general anesthetic in which the woman is put into a medically induced deep sleep for the surgery.
3 Bradycardia means slowing of the heartbeat.
4 The German is Gestell often translated as 'enframing' and re-interpreted by A. Mitchell. In Mitchell's opinion, Heidegger intended the notion of Gestell not as surrounding and framing like water is surrounded and enclosed in a well, but of a gathering; a 'placing and putting' movement of technology (Heidegger, 1994/2012). For the purposes of this thesis, I use Mitchell's interpretation which is congruent with the data analysis.
5 A ventouse birth involves a vacuum extractor instrument that's attached to the baby's head by suction. It is type of instrumental birth to assist the birth by pulling, guiding, and sometimes repositioning the head so that it comes out the birth canal.
6 The Goddess Sophia is the 'Mother of All' or 'Wisdom'. In Gnostic tradition Sophia was born of silence. She is the feminine figure of the human soul, coexisting as the feminine aspect of Divinity (Matthews, 2001).

References

De Leon, J. (2005). *Dance and Stillness*. Auckland: Faculty of Health and Environmental Studies, AUT University.

Gadamer, HG. (1960/1975). *Truth and Method*. New York: Seabury.

Heidegger, M. (1927/1962). *Being and Time*. New York: Harper.

Heidegger, M. (1971/2001). *Poetry, Language, Thought*. New York: HarperCollins.

Heidegger, M. (1993/1954). The question concerning technology. In: D.F. Krell, ed., *Basic Writings*. New York: Harper Collins, pp. 311–341.

Heidegger, M. (1995). *The Fundamental Concepts of Metaphysics: World, Finitude, Solitude*. Bloomington IN: Indiana University Press.

Matthews, C. (2001). *Sophia: Goddess of Wisdom, Bride of God*. London: Theosophical Publishing House.

Parse, R.R. (1997). Joy–sorrow: A study using the Parse research method. *Nursing Science Quarterly*, 10, pp. 80–87.

Rethmann, P. (2006). On presence. In: J. Goulet and B.G.M., eds, *Extraordinary Anthropology*. London: University of Nebraska Press, pp. 36–52.

Smith, Q. (1981). On Heidegger's theory of moods. *The Modern Schoolman*, 58, pp. 211–235.

Spiers, J. (2019). Authentic caring: An Australian experience. In: J. Hoffman, P. Blessinger and M. Makhanya, eds, *Strategies for Facilitating Inclusive Campuses in Higher Education: International Perspectives on Equity and Inclusion*. Bingley, UK: Emerald Publishing Limited, pp. 31–40.

5   Joy as spatial and embodied

The previous chapter made visible a phenomenon named 'joy at birth'. Now we turn to how such joy is revealed as an embodied and spatial experience. The distinctions of place and space and material body and embodied joy are explored. These spatial and embodied qualities of joy at birth are then shown as conjoined meaningful lived-experiences.

Embodied joy

Participants speak of how the experience of birth is felt bodily often throwing them into feelings that are physically intense:

> I'm just moved because it's in those times where you just get to be a bit more human and soak up the awe. To be honest when you get that rush of emotion from the parents, I get the little tears well up and I sort of have to sniff them back and focus on doing the stitches and medical things! That happens often actually that I have to pull myself back into the medical stuff. I don't know exactly what happens in that moment. I can't remove myself from those beautiful experiences and enjoying it. It is more than the medical stuff to me it's spiritual as well, 'cos it seems so special, if it were all just chance, I wouldn't be touched so closely.
>
> (Brenda – obstetrician)

Brenda narrates an account of recent births and describes how she is physically affected as a clinician. She speaks of an intense mood at birth that comes from nowhere and everywhere that is embodied. She is touched physically as she marvels at the mysterious nature of birth. This is far more than a physiological event. For Brenda birth is an event infused with ineffable mystery into which she is thrown as she sniffs back tears. She finds herself attuned in awe to something special and responds in an embodied way.

Smile all over your body

Participants describe a sense of totalising embodied joy irrupting at birth. Tui [a grandmother] describes this beautifully:

There was this great wonderful feeling and I was just kind of in it. It's like having a smile all over your body. It is a smile that just kind of spreads and doesn't go away. It feels like your whole body's just smiling. It's a time in which there is a very peaceful joy. A feeling of being part of the world too, like the world is real and you're really in it. You're right there and you're right in it.

Smiling all over, the smile spreading and remaining; the story, too, invokes a smile. Down to the last fibre of her physical body, Tui is joyful. Her body sighs and smiles in pleasure at the birth. This is an ontological experience. Wrapped in a warm blanket of bliss, she is touched deeply.

Tears of joy

Karl [father] similarly experiences the moments of his son's birth with tears of joy:

When his head started to come out, I could feel a sort of excitement rising in the room, the midwives began moving around … I could see them all getting zingy and the sense of excitement was in the room, everyone was getting excited. I could feel that it was happening, and I remember at times feeling soft waves of tearfulness, the realisation that wow, it really was happening, it is really real the baby is here, arriving. The soft tears were thankfulness and gratitude to God, to the universe and life for producing the moment.

Karl is aware of the increased midwife activity and a mood of inescapable excitement that spreads. His son was finally coming. He is bodily overcome by the shared nature of excitement and relief; there is overwhelming joy in the space that shows itself in embodied waves of soft tearfulness and gratitude. Amy [mother] describes these tearful first moments after birth:

I remember feeling very teary very quickly when she was out. Like an intense wave of emotion. The emotion was love. It was a pretty whole-body experience It was just this feeling of reverence and I'm like "Wow", it's happened, a wow moment, having all your hands up [hands rose] to be a witness to the wonder, that spark of preciousness and to see it in that moment.

There is a sense of tremendous fulfilment and achievement, a bubbling up of love, and tearful exuberant joy as the newborn arrives amidst them.

Breath

Lorna [mother] speaks of how the moment of birth are so overwhelming that her breath is taken away:

The love is so overwhelming that it could stop your breath. I just never, never let anyone hurt her. Just to protect her my girl! It is an all-encompassing love. Very special, very special precious jewel.

This sudden and intense change in mood at the birth is such that it alters the breathing of those present. Anehera [midwife] recognises and facilitates this shift:

> I just like to give them all that moment … just to realise she's just given birth and for everyone just to take a breath. I give everybody the chance to catch their breath while I am drying the baby. Allowing the baby to fill their lungs up. Taking time … the baby is still all curled up trying to take their first breath. I like babies being able to take a big breath and have a cry and let everyone know they're here.

This tells of the preciousness of those initial moments embodied through breath. There is a feeling that everyone needs to take pause for the enormity of what happens in the time of birth. The intensity of the event is over. There is relief, and everyone in the room takes a breath along with the baby. The breathing seemingly breathes life into an awakening joy to which they turn collectively. As the baby fills his/her lungs for the first time a sound is made and when those there in that moment hear that first breath and cry – joy arrives:

> When the baby was here, the elation, relief and joy flooded in and it didn't matter who's there, or if the lights are on, the baby came out crying and went straight to the parents, 'just be there', then everything was alright.
>
> (Simone – midwife)

These immediate moments are a time of joy as the baby announces itself through those first sounds of life. These are significant kinaesthetic moments wherein all the senses are heightened. The sensory impact of a baby taking its first breath and crying awakens joy from within at relief of a safe birth. Tensions and anxieties evaporate in the sound of new life. This auditory experience reveals more of the sudden overwhelming sensory pleasure of joy at birth.

Seeing joy

There are many visual images at birth. Often there is an intense knowing upon seeing others in new ways and seeing the baby for the first time which often brings joy. The visual expression of joy is captured by Amy's [mother] story of seeing her partner's face:

> One of the strongest memories of that whole experience actually was seeing Bill's face in those precious early moments after Ellie was born. Those seconds after Ellie was born and seeing Bill's face and the emotion on his face; it was all just pouring out, relief probably, but also happiness and amazement. I felt like his face reflected exactly what I was feeling. It was amazing to see it, because you can't see yourself. It was amazing to have that mirror and I'm sure my face looked exactly the same.

Amy describes experiencing the mood through the mirror of Bill's facial expressions: emotions of relief, happiness, and amazement "pouring out". This memory is central to Amy's experience and speaks again of the collective nature of the experience at birth. Simone [midwife] similarly captures this shared embodied joy through seeing the first glimpse of the baby:

> When I saw the hair of the baby, suddenly there is this flooding in of joy. It's like the mood suddenly changed in the whole room; the mood changed totally. We were all there around the birthing pool and the baby just emerged and her partner reached down and picked the baby up out of the water and it was calm; that connection between everybody there is beautiful. Including me, what a privilege!

Joy can be delayed but it is in the 'seeing' that joy irrupts. Simone speaks about a caesarean section:

> ...the elation isn't there immediately but from seeing the baby comes the joy.

The visual impact, not just of her baby, but of the physical environment is revealed in Cathy's description of seeing her baby for the first time following hospital induction of labour:

> When I looked at him, I felt in awe. I was in awe. I was in awe that I'd given birth; amazed that we'd gone through it. I remember thanking Dina [midwife], just saying: 'come look, come look at him'. That was the point that dawn had just broken, and the fog was covering the building, the new day had just broken, and he was lying on me. It was pretty magical.
>
> (Cathy – mother)

There is such a sense of joy and connection in this story. The view of the sky through the hospital window infuses the occasion in a meaningful visual way. The visual is ontological as the seeing penetrates into poetic symbolic timeless realms. Seeing warms and cheers the heart turning her to joy. Joy has a look when watched. Marie [midwife] speaks of how a woman is enthralled by repeatedly seeing the video of her rapid birth on the toilet floor of the hospital:

> Her perception was that it was wonderful and therefore it was lovely. It was the perfect birth for her. She kept going on about how wonderful it was and the joy of being able to see it not just the memory of it. She kept looking at the video and seeing herself looking down in joy at her baby. This woman had a look of joy on her face.

The joy becomes visible in the mother's face as she embodies joy at the birth of her baby.

Joy's fragrance

Joy at birth seemingly also brings with it its own fragrance. Along with seeing the sense of smell is heightened:

> He smelt good. I was like, mmm, he smells lovely. *'Ahhh, hello, you'*, I can remember the smell of both of them [looking at her two children in the room during the interview].
>
> (Lorna – mother)

Olfactory memory of her newborn's scent re-rekindles a warming sense of joy and brings a smile to Lorna as she remembers each of her baby's fragrances. The sensual communication between mother and baby is instant and sweet, adding to the lived-experience of the initial joyful meeting. I am reminded how the scent of a newborn connects to tenderness and a string of memories invoking a warm bodily sense of joy in me as I sit here and type. Smell has both physical and ontological dimensions.

Joy as tactile

Closely connected to smell is the tactile experience, an intra-corporal joining associated with profound release into joy:

> As soon as he came out there was this rush of love, maybe within seconds, he came out and he went straight on me. Just looking at him, just touching him, the smell of him. The eye contact, just looking at you, almost like we're just both seeing each other for the first time but we've known each other for a long time. He knew who I was, and I knew who he was. It was so special. A feeling of *'I will protect you with my life.'*
>
> (Lorna – mother)

Lorna describes how each of her senses is part of the bonding process and central to joy at birth. There is a sense that the physical touching of a baby invokes a certain mood that touches participants. Brenda [obstetrician] also speaks about the special moment of touching a baby at caesarean section:

> As soon as I reach in and can touch the baby, I feel excited as I get to be the very first one to touch it! I reach in and it's like this first connection with the baby. I have to feel exactly how it's lying. As soon as the hand goes in and touches the baby there is a transition to something. It's hard because I'm constantly balancing between the medical bit and the connection. In that instance I'm focused on me and getting the baby out safely (smiles). It is a privilege.
>
> (Brenda)

When Brenda touches the baby for the first time a special connection is made. In that moment an intimate relationship comes into being between her and the unborn baby. The baby and Brenda move together, akin to an instantaneous spell cast on tactile contact, Brenda is warmed by the memory and smiles; it is a special and thrilling moment in her work. The obstetric concerns and responsibilities juxtapose with the intimate human connection between doctor and unborn infant. How does the baby bring forth such powerful changes? This first physical touch is significant, initiating a profound sense of spiritual connection in otherwise medical situations.

I am reminded that to touch is to be touched (Merleau-Ponty, 1962/2002); a shared communication through the medium of touch. When participants touch the baby, they also feel themselves being touched. Thus, touch unlike seeing and hearing, involves a double relation. Touch distinguishes us from objects as the body senses itself. The tactile contact seemingly transcends this bodily aspect and speaks of an ontological touching. Touching, in the Heideggerian sense, involves worlds touching. Conversely, two world-less objects, like a chair and a wall, can touch each other physically yet cannot touch ontologically. Human beings or Daseins thus touch each other physically and ontologically. Dasein is not merely intra-worldly but inextricably one in the 'worlds'. As such participants are Being-in-the-world and therefore always touched and touching the baby's body feels separate but is paradoxically not separate.

Chocolate feeling

Touch at birth reveals a sense of connection as participants literally 'body the experience'; they are touched in physical and ontological ways that feel joyful. Through the touching and all the other sensorial experiences, participants become the world-of-birth. Tui [grandmother] beautifully illuminates this as she speaks of a 'chocolate feeling' when all the senses are flooded with delight:

> A couple of days after the birth when his bowels hadn't moved, and my daughter was really worried about that she suddenly realised that she loved this baby so much that she couldn't stand it to happen to him. So that was great, she got the chocolate feeling. When the bond was there straight away with the last grandchild's birth I stood back. It was like, the world's right.

Tui points to the importance of that initial bonding through holding and touching that embodies joy and love. The world is not right until the newborn is touched and bonds with someone. Tui believes that the moment of birth is privative without this and is relieved once her daughter attunes to that feeling. The bonding feeling appears essential to the nature of birth and significant in its absence.

Tui's wisdom reflects what others have said about the deleterious effects when there is lack of bonding. Perhaps there is a shared cocktail of hormones at birth inducing something special that Tui describes, as a 'chocolate feeling', a falling in love with the newborn. How this occurs is unclear, yet it is part of Tui's lived-experience at birth. For Tui touch is more than bodily contact. It is about being touched and is constitutive of the experience of mood at birth. The birthing woman's physiological changes may or may not be shared but Tui points to how a special feeling spreads out regardless. The chocolate feeling evokes a sudden and welcomed delicious, sensual, sweet embodied joyful experience.

Embodied suddenness

The sudden nature of this embodied reaction is described further by Lorna [mother]:

> I felt very shaky, like I was actually physically shaking like a leaf. I also had that sense of relief. I had done a good job and gave myself a pat on the back. I was really proud that I'd had a homebirth and that it was really calm, and everything went well.

Lorna speaks of a mixture of experiences at birth. Relief is evident at the birth process being completed safely. There is physical shock as her body reacts then adjusts to the suddenness of events. The physical experience floods her and she is inseparable from the joy. Cathy [mother] also speaks of the sudden changed mood once the birth is over:

> The birth itself is different too; to having him on you at the end. It's something altogether different. The birth is the hard work and once he's on your chest it's the beginning; the birth was the end, and this is the beginning. They're not one and the same.

Cathy describes how the intra-corporal contact with the newborn suddenly turns her to an irrupting joy. It seems as if there are layers of emotional states, like happiness and anxiety, as well as corporal/visceral aspects that flow into an intensely joyful embodied experience. Lorna continues:

> I was just really delighted to meet him that sense of meeting him properly. All the time I've been carrying him and growing him and keeping him safe from harm and now he is out into the world and there was this intense rush of love, just so happy to meet him finally. So much happiness.

The moment(s) of birth seem to reveal something else; an overwhelming passion of love for the newborn whatever the circumstances. Lorna had birthed a 32-week breech baby in hospital following an ambulance transfer from a remote rural location.

Joy is an embodied experience at birth

Joy at birth is experienced through the totality of bodily senses. The nature of touching, holding, smelling, seeing, and hearing, something captivating and attracting in the experience of birth mood is revealed. Powerful sensual and ontological responses reveal a joy at birth. According to Merleau-Ponty

(1962/2002), the body is the medium of all perception. Van Manen (1990) explains this as "... we are always bodily in the world" (103). Embodied joyful experience is both the material body and the living experiencing body. Body and experience are an inseparable togetherness,

> ... down to the last muscle fibre and hidden molecule of hormones belongs to existence including our senses ... we are not able to see because we have eyes; rather, we can only have eyes because, according to our basic nature, we are beings who can see.
>
> (Heidegger, 2001: 232)

We sensorially experience birth not because we have physical senses but because we are beings that feel. Joy at birth is not determined by sensorial experiences only; it is those experiences and more. Heidegger does not condone the 'splitting' up of the human being into body-soul-spirit, conceiving of ourselves as a unity of this tripartite notion. Instead Heidegger challenges us to think in a different way by changing the word 'body' to a verb, contending that to live experience is to body experience. The existential experience of embodied joy has shown how the world of birth reaches out to participants due to the spatiality of the body and how participants reach out towards birth attuning as they do to birth as embodied experience. I observed in my field notes that participants are bodily attuning to joy at birth in shared reciprocity:

> Moving and being moved
> holding and being held
> touching and being touched
> feeling and being felt
> seeing and being seen
> hearing and being heard

Spatial joy

Embodied joy cannot be understood in isolation. Participants equally point to a special space in which embodied joy at birth experience unfolds. This is an attuned spatial joy, a feeling space which is embodied. A place of birth is not defined as hospital or home, but rather is significant as a safe place to birth, a friendly place, a warm place, a noisy room, a cold room, an exposed room. Place may be the hospital physical environment, yet it is the space that is meaningful within that place. As such birth places open up meaningful spaces in which birth is experienced and disclosed differently.

Being-in sacred space

Amy [mother] describes her experience of birth space:

> It was both beauty and potent. The different expressions of love were there in this room; there's this smiling at each other, lots of physical contact, lots

of holding, lots of space. There's that real sense of knowing and feeling. Being aware of each other. Love for me relates to those around me as it's more tangible when it's reflected back at me. The fundamental basis at birth was being in this sacred space.

For Amy there is a sense of connectedness that is constitutive of birth space; a quality of feeling-space. She speaks of the space of birth as a field of gathering, a space that holds and invites an experience of tangible love. It is an interconnected sense of knowing and awareness of others that gestures a relational space at birth. The experience of her daughter's birth engenders pinnacle awareness. The joy she encounters is through her body, her own emotional world, and those around her within that shared space. There is a sense of nurture, honouring, loving, and delight in this story as she speaks of an open and sacredly enriched space that is not privative. For Amy this is a space that is enjoyed in its wholeness and completeness, a space in which she enjoys dwelling.

Amy had planned a homebirth but had been transferred to hospital with labour dystocia. She found herself in the clinical hospital environment yet the joyful space at birth opened a feeling of nurturing; not an alien, hostile, hospital room. Amy experiences the hospital in ways that she may not have done on a different day. Heidegger refers to this aspect of spatiality as 'directionality' (Heidegger, 1927/1962).[1] This refers to how space can be perceived differently according to situation and ways of attuning.

The notion of feeling-space is both separated yet one and the same as physical-place. This feeling-space is experienced as a space infused by a spirit of Being and attunement that discloses safety, belonging, and loving care. Amy's experience of dwelling at birth within a particular feeling-space is pleasing, homely, and inviting. To be in such sacred space, as Amy names it, is to be at once attuned joyfully; a joy that is at once the melding of space and place itself to which one belongs and feels at home as place and space become inseparable.

Simone [midwife] too describes being with-in a sacred birth space:

I felt in awe and just so privileged to be there but not interrupt it, I just kept the door closed and nobody else came in the room at all in the hospital. Outside the rooms a lot is going on; hustle and bustle and bright lights and talk around the board of whom is in the birthing rooms. There is a lot of activity and technology. In the room we could create our own space, a sacred space.

Simone describes a sacred space in which labour and birth occur. There is something outside of that sacred space existing in the physical room. This sacred space is described as open but small and warm, a space that is calm and devoid of disturbing or unsettling activity. In this intimate quiet space something magical is emerging, the deepest tenderness and connection of all present moving as one. Outside this special meaningful space is the hospital and its related '*hustle and bustle and bright lights*', the antithesis of the sensitive mood in the room where this labour and birth is unfolding. Outside lacks the personal and sensitive nature of this gentle attuned sacred space.

Dwelling in a bubble

Amy [mother] describes this space as being in a 'bubble':

> The three of us kind of like huddled together, just kind of felt this intense sense of togetherness. It was like in the room around us there were lots going on because the obstetrician had been in and people were coming and they would stand in the corner, and there was a whole team of them. I don't really remember that as I was too busy. Ellie and I and Pete were in our own little bubble then.

There is the sense of an inside and outside of attuned space. The bubble seems to provide a protective gossamer-like layer around them, affording an intimacy and calmness. Within this bubble Amy and Pete are busy meeting and bonding with their new baby whilst all outside concerns evaporate. The attuned joyous space reveals itself as having boundaries.

Being-in and being-out of birth's felt-space

Tui [grandmother] describes the full potency of being within this felt boundary space:

> There is something about being there. I think you have to be ... you have to feel it. Some of my children have had babies and rung me afterwards. But it's not the same. The grandchildren that I have been there for their births, I'm much closer to, that bond is stronger. It's certainly stronger when I've been there for the birth.

Tui highlights a significant attribute of the experience of spatial joy at birth by distinguishing being there in the space and not being there. According to Tui, one needs to be in the room, the physical location where the birth occurs. Otherwise it is simply not the same. It would appear to lose its potency. Tui compares being at the births of grandchildren and not being there, expressing that it is not as strong a lived-experience of being there in the place where it happens. She then shares the consequences of not being in the place of birth. Significantly, Tui has noticed that she is more closely bonded to the grand-children whose births she has been able to experience Being-in the joyous space.

It is unclear what proximity is required to be touched and affected by joy at birth. However, from my field notes I recall that material objects are not a barrier:

> I just went to see a student on the birthing unit. The staff said she was in a room with a labouring woman and that it was okay to go in. I approached the door, and then stopped before I knocked, I pressed my ear to the door and the silence was deafening, then a series of deep guttural breathes. I

retreated and went to my car. I have been touched by the space of birth and I find myself smiling as I organise to drive home, everything looks sparkly somehow.

(In the car park of the hospital – November 2011)

Although I was not physically in the room, the birth space reached out to me and I, in turn, reached into it; I was touched enough to be concerned not to disrupt a special feeling-space and yet at the same time experienced some of its uplifting essence. There appears to be a fluidity of a joyful feeling-space that discloses a communal sensitivity and tact. It seems that something about the space of birth is special, regardless of physical aspects. Simone [Midwife] describes this well:

> Every time I go into a hospital, it's very clinical, sterile and clean, yet there's still a part of me that says, *'even though this is a hospital, this is a sacred place because life is brought into the world here, new life emerges here'*, therefore there has to be something special about that place, something sacred.

The place of birth appears to open a meaningful space that engages and holds us. I am reminded of how parents proudly point out the stained carpet on a home visit and say that was where he/she was born, 'right there!'

I am also reminded in the debates about place of birth and how they can infer exclusionary moves. Attachment to a particular place can lead to separation and exclusion of others through political, cultural, and traditional dictates, for example, the birthing room can be protected from unwanted others such as fathers. Although place of birth opens spaces which are imbued with meanings that differ according to circumstances (i.e. temporal and sociocultural contexts), it appears that joy at birth overrides exclusionary border debates and disputes. Joy at birth can disclose a special space even in an operating theatre at the time of birth. Even when there are no established relationships, as often the case when others arrive to assist at an emergency, joy is just there. Rather than being exclusory birth's feeling space involves an experience of gathering and a sense of belonging. It seems plausible to assume that birth is always significant wherever and however it unfolds. This is not to deny that interventions do not and cannot alter the mood at birth, because as the previous chapter revealed they can.

Space opens in unexpected places

Birth also happens quickly and in unexpected places. In my pre-understandings interview I recalled experiencing a birth in the front seat of a truck:

> The birth was in the car park outside the rural birth unit. There is pandemonium as emergency services and medical practitioners arrive. Meanwhile my head pops into the birth space to reveal a mother trying to prise her newborn out of knickers smiling as she does so at the wriggling baby. We laughed, discovered the sex of her baby and enjoyed the birth.

Few would choose to birth in a vehicle, yet even such a birth can open a feeling-space. The birthing 'space' in the truck is enjoyed whilst others panicked at the 'place' where it was unfolding. Birth can be unplanned and sudden which can lead to unexpected situations; yet, joy is still possible. Marie [midwife] speaks of an unplanned vaginal birth after caesarean section in a car without any midwife or medical assistance to hand:

> I had a woman who went into labour who had had two previous CSs [caesarean sections]. I suggested she goes to the nearest hospital because we were not near to each other, and she said no, I will just go home. Anyway, she phones again a few hours later to say she wants to push. The husband was panicking, and her two sons were in the car too. I just said just keep the baby warm, maintain skin to skin don't worry about the cord. I could hear the baby crying so I knew all was fine. 2 and half hours later they arrived at the hospital. There was hilarity around because something unexpected had happened; just laughter and joy. Everything had turned out so unexpectedly. Despite all the risks and drama, it was a sense of triumph; even with her knickers on.

The unplanned "place" for this birth is flooded by celebration and jollity that discloses the specialness of the feeling-space that opened. It appears that physical environment of birth can fade as a special birth space opens. In that opening the physical birthplace can become symbolic and integrated as in Cathy's dawn birth story and Marie's story of the woman that had a car birth without midwife or medical assistance. There can even be a sense of hilarity at birth, as in the truck birth.

Feeling space as opening

Whatever and however birth unfolds those present at that moment are thrown into a feeling-space that invokes a response, even if the response is to turn away. Karl [father] describes a special attuning that he can turn to and enter but not generate. A feeling-space that exists whether he is aware of it or not that requires a turning towards, openness, and engagement:

> There was flow within the atmosphere to connect the heart and mind with that intention of the spiritual realm. The birth process needed to be in a spiritual flow. You are in the flow you are not generating it. You are opening yourself to an ever-present flow that exists. By opening to it you begin to feel it and become aware of it and you can perceive it more.

There is a sense of flowing that takes him into that space once he turns towards it and feels its specialness, which he names 'spiritual flow'. Karl's description is one of movement that speaks of a quality of dynamic mystical space and numinous experience. It is plausible that attuning to spatial joy at birth acts as a doorway to how differences and possibilities can be revealed. Although birth 'place' and birth 'space' seem distinctly different, they intertwine. As place and space become conflated, they become a clearing in which awareness of birth's significance shows itself. The birth space revealed by Karl is disclosed by wonder and awe. Being thrown into the experience of being there at birth seemingly confronts us with a mystery and turning towards and being in a spatial joy at birth is felt as 'magical'.

Simone [midwife] describes this magical space as addictive:

> I think it can be a bit addictive! When someone calls me, I feel elation for them really! That there is an awaited baby – this baby that's been growing inside them is ready, has decided to come. It's still that same feeling, even when it is complicated … it can be addictive, addiction to joy can lead to a lot of sacrifices in my family. It's very fulfilling and I have got a little bit addicted to that joy.

There is a magnetically captivating quality to the joy at birth that claims Simone. This hints at a seductive even intoxicating quality of the space at birth. Tui [grandmother] adds:

> That joy and that feeling of love is like you're absolutely intoxicated! This is the highest feeling and each time afterwards I would think; I really want to be a midwife! I want this all the time, this really high intoxicated feeling. I want to hold onto that intoxicating feeling for all it's worth. I was high for maybe a week after that. I was just kind of walking around in a cloud, smiling to everyone, loving the world. I think with all the births I've been at there is always this lasting feeling that lasts for a long time afterwards.

Tui craves to be in this cherished space for as long as possible and enjoys its intoxicating quality. She is helplessly drawn into this feeling and carried away by the intense pleasure of being in a spatial joy opened at birth. There is a sense of surrender to a power that literally detaches her from everyday preoccupations with past and future, a sense of dislocation from time. Birth demands her full attention. It drags her into the moment and describes a strong and lingering 'feel good factor'. There is no fear in her narrative. She craves to be with-in this joy and be carried away by its mystery.

Birth space is a meaningful feeling-space that is perceived with delight, appreciation, and connectedness. Birth-space is something altogether different from the everyday spaces of our lives – it is a profound opening to something more. This is a space filled with something extraordinary in quality that touches participants profoundly. It is a revered and honoured space that holds a sense of the miraculous. I noted in several post-interview field notes how the notion of privilege comes through strongly and sense of wonder and miraculous nature of being in the space at birth. Marie [midwife] articulates this well:

> I look on my life as a midwife as being very blessed, privileged always to be invited into this amazing journey. I am somehow renewed by my midwifery. I believe that now as I plan to retire, I will treasure those years of being invited into the family. I am always 'drawn', I hope I never lose that.

Marie feels fortunate to be there and be part of this event and is humbled by its auspiciousness. To be in that spatial joy at birth discloses her concern with authentic ways of being in the world of birth. She dwells in an opening of genuine concern that releases her from the dictates of the One: the dictatorship of policies, guidelines, mass-media, and professional politics. Spatial joy at birth is wholly different to the place of one's identity and everyday professional and personal concerns.

Spatial joy would seem to hint at a coming home at birth. This homecoming points back to the primordial questionability of being that has always already been there; a space in which being-towards-life is played out. Birth-space is perhaps a play of the places in which birth unfolds, for *anywhere* can enact the sacred at birth and the joy that discloses such potential. It is not only the quiet intimate homebirth that opens joyful sacred spaces at birth. The place where a baby is born becomes sanctified as a feeling space opens, even in the front of a truck joy at birth can awaken. Maternity hospitals too can be sanctified places and meaning filled spaces where joy and birth arrives. What appears to matter is turning towards the dynamic experience of joy and allow ourselves to be deeply touched by it ontologically.

Joy, anxiety and sorrow in the birth space

Joy at birth is dynamic within it resides an inherent sense of movement. It may be that we need to traverse anxiety prior to arriving at joy when birth is complete. We have seen how birth is constituted of suddenness, surprise, overwhelm, and change. Perhaps the joy spoken of at birth is fundamental to the experience concurrent with an ever-present anxiety? Is it through such anxiety, as Heidegger contends, that something more authentic is revealed in "unshakable joy" and "bliss of astonishment" (Heidegger, 1995). Perhaps joy and anxiety are entwined and fundamental to our experiences at birth providing the intensity and magnitude of the occasion. There is a sense that the turbulence of mood undergoes a continual metamorphosis that culminates as an awakened intense overwhelming moment of joy that is felt bodily and spatially at birth. Fear can move to love, anxiety to relief, and relief to joy – this movement can be quick as a flash or evolve gently as the occasion unfolds. What is evident is how these moods lead to nurturing, safe-guarding, and sheltering of the newborn. These co-existing and dynamic moods seem integral to the lived-experience of joy at birth. Todnes and Galvin (2010) describe such dynamism as part of an existential theory of wellbeing potential that leads us to feeling home. The dynamic nature of moods in the birth-space maybe leading us home to something existentially significant.

There are certainly situations when joy at birth is not awakened; times when sorrow awakens at birth. Simone [midwife] remembers a maternal death and the juxtaposition of being confronted with life and death:

> I think of a time when I felt this sacred space was disrupted most was the death of a mother. The relationship between the woman and her husband and the intimacy and the anticipation of the new life coming … [Long pause] the

mother went to the bathroom and didn't come back [long pause] then it was just like white lightening and bright lights and people ... [cries] I just didn't think it would come back like this [crying]. But when you contextualise it in relation to the beauty of birth and new life and then death enters. The joy was there because the baby was coming; there was no hint that kind of thing was going to happen ... the baby could've died, but it didn't. It's almost like it wasn't the baby's time to die, [whispers] but it was the mother's time. I did not really think on the baby then but now when I look back, it is a miracle.

A deep feeling of concern and connectedness is revealed in this sad experience. The absence of joy is obvious as sorrow awakens. The potential for joy dies with the death of the mother. Death disrupts the sacred birth space and Simone is deeply upset. Mood in this story is one of sorrow; a tragedy that is embodied in tears and silence. Joy is covered over by sadness, yet a trace of joy remains. When Simone reflects, she sees the survival of the baby as a miracle that was somehow hidden in the tragic events. In her re-calling joy awakens amidst the sorrow. Even in a stillbirth there is something both sad and joyful. I professionally experienced a 34-week stillbirth in my own midwifery caseload practice:

> It was sad to be called to this stillbirth, it was so calm, so family warming somehow special and holy, yes it was still a sacred moment.
>
> (Reflective diary)

There is a deep sense of reverence and care that touches ontologically at birth regardless of outcome. Death at birth feels dissolute compared with what may have been. This again points to the significance of birth in all circumstances and how respect and tenderness for the spatial and embodied qualities of the experience are important to acknowledge. Those at birth when there is tragedy attune in ways that attempt to reconcile the irreconcilable. There appears to be hidden depths to the meaning of birth however and in whatever way it unfolds even if joy seems to be challenged.

Birth engenders care and concern and it can be assumed that all those there at birth wish for the occasion to be joyful. The potency of attuned space at birth and how this reaches and touches our deepest aspirations and desires to care are revealed further in times of loss. To care, according to Heidegger, is our facticity, our way of Being-in-the-world that constitutes who we are as a whole. How birth attunes, spatially and bodily, matters. Those present at birth are consistently inspired to safeguard and shelter an embodied and spatial joy. Joy is meaningful and significant and discloses how in embodied mood and attuned space participants are focused on Being-towards-birth collectively through their care and concern. Carol [obstetrician] reveals her deep concern about babies born into socio-economic difficulties:

> There is just insecurity about the family having this new baby. I sit on the perinatal mortality and morbidity [meeting] for this region and I can see that the still born birth and neonatal death rate is high among these young women

who have very little support, very little economic support. I see those babies being born into that scenario and it makes me sad. This makes me feel sad at the time of the birth if I can see that or know about the situation.

This brings into focus that not all births are contextually happy events. The feeling-space at such births is often sad for Carol as she feels concern for how that baby's life will unfold after having been born into this situation. For Carol such circumstances lack the joy associated with birth, the birth lacks the openness to the potential of new life. Possibilities are hidden in the milieu of social risks of what may happen. The significance of joy at birth is further highlighted in such concern when it seemingly retreats in shadow.

Does such sadness and concern reflect the significance of birth that spurns us to care? Carol's concern reflects van Manen's (2002) care-as-worry "the more I care for this other, the more I worry and the stronger my desire to care" (270). Van Manen weaves the interpretation of care and worry together revealing the experience that Carol describes; a concern that carries the "burden of responsibility" (277) that van Manen compares to a chronic condition of worrying. There is a recurrent theme in which joy at birth is experienced differently when there are challenging aspects at birth. Yet the experience at the time of birth always opens an attuned space and is always bodily felt somehow.

The significance of birth-space and the embodied nature of this experience may hold greater than assumed importance. Re-calling the experience of joy at birth re- opens that joyous space. I, too, moved into a joy filled feeling-space along with the participants as I listened to their stories, feeling physically stirred again and again in the reading and analysis. Participants often became positively attuned as they narrated their stories. They entered a spatial and embodied joy made visible through their tears, laughter, smiling, and touching. There was tangible pleasure at the remembrance of precious moments that hinted at the profundity of potent and tender experiences:

> The birth is just the launching pad for this person (looks at his son) so you want to provide a really good experience as he comes into the world, so he has a good impression of this place (tears in his eyes). That he can feel loved and supported, nurtured and it's a very firm foundation to grow and to become a good person. It is a benefit for all humanity to have as many good people on the planet as possible.
>
> (Karl – father)

Embodied joy reawakened as Karl narrates. There is a sense of acknowledgement of overwhelming responsibility that brings him to tears of joy as he gazes upon his newborn son. Significant long-lasting impressions from the direct experience of dwelling with-in an embodied spatial joy at birth are revealed in Karl's story.

Birth experiences are consistently reported as fulfilling, absorbing, and meaningful. Birth is a powerful event that acts as a rite of passage bringing responsibility and change of life roles. Life feels different after the birth and leaves those there at birth opened to possibilities previously not considered. There is a sense of a lasting on-going deepening happiness, growing connection, and love for the newborn, a baby that appears to be centre stage in this feeling-space and embodied lived-experience. It is an occasion of caring and concerned ways of being.

Joy discloses the world-of-birth through embodied and spatial ways. Yet, without Dasein (open engagement in the situation) such embodied and spatial interpreted experiences would not be possible. The sacred-space at birth is opened due to Dasein's Being-there. It is the Being-there which opens sacred joyful space at birth. In other words that moment of birth 'is' Dasein openly engaged in that world. The world of birth is not something that is only known in a sensory manner but is presented to participants through the facticity[2] of their always already attunement. To be spatially and bodily attuned to joy at birth is to be Dasein thrown into that occasion. Dasein is Being-in and at once becoming the joyous space and embodied joy. Spatial and embodied joy are constituent aspects of joy at birth that are in the interiority of each other.

Conclusion

This chapter has brought together the existential notions of attuned joy at birth as embodied-spatial phenomenon. The constitutive notions have revealed 'something' about how joy at birth is experienced, something, as Heidegger alludes to that is "… so strange that [we] cannot grasp its primordial character at all". Through the distinctions of embodied and spatial experiences, birth mood reveals textual dynamic lived-experiences that culminate as an irrupting moment of joy at the time of birth. These distinctions in experiential terms are felt as place and felt space co-existing as equally important parts of the whole phenomenon inseparable from the experiential embodied joy at birth.

Something special about being at birth has been uncovered; a profound experience wherein the arrival of a new human being invites and pulls participants into joy that is embodied and spatial. By bringing to language the lived-experience of joy as spatial and embodied, new horizons of understanding have opened up that point towards others still to be uncovered. The phenomenon is far from complete and other existential notions require examination. The next chapter uncovers how others gather nearer at the time of birth, revealing the phenomenon 'joy at birth' further.

Notes

1 Heidegger's notion of spatiality is possible only on the basis of Dasein always Being-in. One of the characteristics of 'Being-in' is directionality. The spatial world of participants is not fixed, and directionality shows how Dasein is always in motion in becoming aware of its 'Being-in' situations in a pre-reflective manner that constantly interprets and reinterprets itself in its thrownness (Heidegger, 1927/1962). Thus, the surrounding world blends and integrates the world of participants; that is to say, the spatial world of participants literally 'worlds' perpetually.

2 Facticity is something that already informs and has been taken up in existence, even if it is overlooked or ignored. Our facticity is our innate qualities and states of being, for example, we are always in one mood or another, we are always somehow thrown into situations – it is who and how we are.

References

Heidegger, M. (1995). *Being and Time*. Oxford: Basil Blackwell.

Heidegger, M. (2001). *Zollikon Seminars: Protocols – Conversations – Letters*. Evanston, IL: Northwestern University Press.

Merleau-Ponty, M. (1962/2002). *The Phenomenology of Perception*. London: Routledge Classics.

Todnes, L. and Galvin, K. (2010). 'Dwelling-mobility': An existential theory of well-being. *International Journal of Studies Health and Well-being*, 5444, pp. 1–6.

van Manen, M. (1990). *Researching Lived Experience*. Ontario: The University of Western Ontario.

van Manen, M. (2002). Care-as-worry, or 'don't worry, be happy'. *Qualitative Health Research*, 12, pp. 262–278.

6 Joy as relational gathering

The previous chapter uncovered the phenomenon of joy at birth as embodied and spatial lived-experience. What began to be revealed is how joy is shared and how we are with one another. There is something about birth which gathers others near into these shared spaces and embodied experiences. Joy at birth as shared experiences and a gathering reveal something significant and meaningful. As we reflect on 'others' at birth we uncover how joy at birth is not individuating but a gathering.

Heidegger explains how mood is not something separate to our coming together: "Attunement is not some being that appears in the soul as an experience, but the way of our Being there with one another" (Heidegger, 1995: 66). Being there at birth with one another as gathering is how we attune in the world-of-birth. This reveals an extraordinary moment in which a relational gathering collectively attunes as the moment of birth draws near.

The moment draws near

In the period leading up to birth anticipatory anxiety often co-exists with an expectation of joy. Sometimes that anxiety can be felt as non-specific dread or fear related to a specific threat. This is not to say these are separate moods but a tension as birth approaches. Lorna [mother] tells of frantic phone calls as she finds herself in strong labour about to birth a premature breech baby:

> I phoned my Mum and my sister because they really wanted to be at the birth. When they told me, the birth was going to happen I quickly get on the phone to my sister. But they missed the birth by ten minutes. I phoned them because I was at the birth of my sister's twins and I really wanted my sister at my birth and I wanted Mum there for support emotionally, mentally, and physically. I just really wanted them there. They told me later how they raced towards the birth worried about what they would find.

Birth gathers and draws others into its special mood. The family members *'raced towards the birth'* worried at the potential outcome but also wanting to be there at the birth. Lorna wants significant others there also; especially as there were issues of risk. Feeling safe and feeling fear play together at this time. The advent of a new human being appears to act as a clarion call to others to be near, to help, to gather, and greet this new baby. They come to birth in anticipation of something special, knowing that birth is significant whatever the outcome; to be at birth is more than everydayness. Lorna's family are compelled and need to be there. The prospect of being at birth is magnetic.

John [father] narrates how birth attracts as a magnet gathering others to itself:

> My Mum came up and she stopped in and just said Hi. They went and Carol's [his wife] sister came, and they were a little bit drunk and provided some entertainment. It was a bit of a family event starting to brew; Carol's sister came also and one of her friends. They all come around because they were excited that baby would soon be here.

John's story illustrates how birth brings relatives and friends close to the place where the baby will be born soon. His family is very excited. There is a sense of intimate inclusiveness yet also a public aspect of this birth drawing others. There is a spirit of growing collectivity as birth approaches; a coming and pulling together as the communal experience unfolds. Feelings of excitement mean others leave their everyday lives to be near. Something momentous is about to happen that draws others into this intimate yet paradoxically public expression of being alive. This is something of significance in the lives of family and friends who are close to the couple and the baby. There is the opportunity for a meaningful encounter with the essence of something special which is alluring. Like a warm fire in winter brings others together around the family hearth so too birth gathers. The magnetic and gathering nature of birth emerges as constitutive of joy's potential.

The joyful anticipation of pregnancy and labour draws to an end amidst concerns for safety and perhaps fear and dread. Then the baby is born. An aspect of the moment of birth is Being-with-others in suddenness, surprise, and movement. These fathers speak of being flooded and soaked by waves of emotions instantly as labour changes to birth:

> Release of pent up energy
>
> (Karl – father)

As Karl's son is born, he feels strong protective feelings and pride as he feels drawn nearer. The sudden thrownness into that first meeting with the newborn surprises as joy irrupts:

> That was a special moment when he just 'flew out'; especially seeing him on Carol [wife]. It was peace, relief and love; we've got a baby, pfoof! He's alive; we've made a human being!
>
> (John – father)

There is a sacred or special quality that seems to come from the baby as it unfurls in the gathering as a feeling of family deepens in that moment. The moment awakens an intensity of joy in its fullness. The dramatic changes can be unsettling as waves of emotions surge through the gathering. This speaks of tenderness and affection towards the baby that is potent, intoxicating, and fascinating to those there. Simone [midwife] describes this significant gathering moment as *"Beautiful naturalness"*. Happiness exudes the gathering in that moment like a light switched on, like a *"universal happiness in the room"* exclaims Simone.

Others have written about how something illuminates at birth, Janet Merewether, Australian birth filmmaker (2013), declares "there is a light that comes into the room when a baby is born"; an observation that mirrors my own midwifery practice experiences. In my original field notes I jotted down a comment by an elder midwifery colleague whilst discussing this study; she pondered, turned to me and said, 'arrr, yes, it is like a drop of stardust when the baby is born'. Carol [obstetrician] feels something distinctive in that moment as *"there is always happiness in the room when the baby arrives"*. For Lorna [mother], these moments are gifting a *"precious jewel"*.

There is a feeling that any sense of duality dissolves in the lightness at birth. The shared attuning to joy is revealed in the tears, smiles, tender touches, hugs, and gentle words that draw the gathering nearer. This is something inescapably shared. Mothers, and others, speak of shared tears suddenly irrupting at the suddenness of birth gathering them closer. The moment of birth that cannot be put into language; an awe beyond spoken words that is difficult to articulate: *"an oooh feeling, a whoa or whoo moment!"* [Diane, midwife]. Lorna [mother], with tears in her eyes, describes this as *"beyond special, a moment of grace"*. This is a sudden ineffable moment that shifts into joyous gathering, holding potential for profound connecting and nearness.

Being near

To be near is also a 'feeling close' and 'felt belonging' to the gathering. Being near to birth, as Pat [mother] describes, is more than being physically present.

> I called my dad as he really wanted to know right away when the baby was born. I left a message on his phone and I felt myself welling-up telling him he is a grandfather [begins to weep] I didn't know where the tears were coming from. [silence while crying].

To be near even in absence was revealed in the stories of how birth gathers. This story speaks of an evolution of relationships and emotional connections. Family dynamics are evident as Pat reaches for the phone to gather her father near into the magic of the moment. Birth gifts the possibility to unite and connect, to deepen family feelings, and relationships. One can imagine the sense of joy the grandfather would have on hearing that his grandson is born safely. Although physically not there he is intimately near to the joy at birth within Pat's tears. To be physically present at the moment of birth is not essential to be part of the gathering. Birth appears to hold participants captive in its gathering power as they draw near. Even if it is only the mother and baby physically there at the moments of birth, the thoughts and feelings of others bring those physically far into nearness.

To be in the world is always and already to be with-other. Ontically it may be possible to die alone but to be born is always to be gathered with-others, even if it is just mother and newborn. In contrast, ontologically we are never alone either at birth or death, others are always near and far (Wojtkowiak and Crowther, 2018). This nearness is not measurable but felt as so near as not to be visible. This distinction of nearness is emphasised by Tui [grandmother] in the familiarity of how family and others gather near:

> My daughter, who was one years old at the time, was between my niece's legs as the baby came out. Once the baby was born, we all went to a communal bath in a different house as we had no bath and had a bath with the baby. There was this lovely parade down the street with this new baby to the communal bath. People were waving out their windows and cheering! I remember feeling just warm and exciting. It was great with everyone there, lots of little kids.

This story reveals a sense of shared jubilation at birth as joy spreads out into the community. Others may not be close physically, but they draw near to birth as a communal event of great significance. The children in the story have an important relationship to the event and belong there in the thick of it, all contributing to the shared joy. The physically deprived circumstances do not appear to spoil this occasion despite lack of resources. The sense of celebration at the mystery and magic of new life gathers them all near in shared joy. Being-with-others at birth lies at the heart of how joy is experienced. Karl [father] emphasises this quality of drawing near further:

> There is a special feeling around birth it is joy, everybody is so happy. When you tell people, you've had a baby people are instantly happy and joyful about it. They are so happy and want to contact you and want to come around, they just want to be around 'it'. You can definitely see it even in other people who are not involved. Even people who you hardly even know it is just 'wow that is just so awesome, congratulations, that is awesome' and I am thinking 'you have hardly spoken to me before!

Karl observes that even others whom he does not know well become ensnared in this net of happiness: "*Everyone is just so happy*" he exclaims. Others respond to the joyous news and want to get as near as they can to the specialness. Karl [father] also speaks of a mesmerising quality just after the birth of his son:

> In that hour after the birth you get mesmerised by the baby. Just totally focused, it is just 'woo' you're just watching and listening, just looking at him. Just focused right in, I was magnetised.

Karl describes the intense experience of meeting his son for the first time as mesmerising, his baby acts like a magnet drawing him. Due to birth's hypnotic qualities and pleasurable feelings others are captured into the gathering. Yet the mood at birth is not always joyful for everyone.

Working together

There is a gathering of others at birth who come together for a variety of purposes. For some turning to joy at birth can be difficult. There are times when some who are present must simply turn away from joy:

> I sometimes feel myself overcome and fight back the tears as I have a job to do.
>
> (Brenda – obstetrician)

Brenda needs to turn from joy in order to do her job. She says she sometimes has to fight being overwhelmed by the gathering mood of the occasion. This signals the intensity and strength in the moment of birth as a potent mood awakens calling all to nearness. Those gathered at birth have different roles and responsibilities despite this special potent quality of the atmosphere. Brenda speaks of facing unknown situations in which she feels little joy due to the anxiety and despair of uncertainty that comes with her role:

> My first thoughts when I was called to the room to assess and help was just about organizing the problem into my head and establishing the most vital information. The midwife had handed information before I entered the room: "*Where is she in labour, how long has she been pushing for and is the baby positioned well. What are the features on the trace, how urgently do we need to act?*" When I first entered the room, it was quite anxious because I entered expecting the worst we've been called in for a problem.

There is an inherent mood of anticipatory anxiety and uncertainty in this story. For Brenda birth brings the potential for life and death. Perhaps she experiences a chronic worrying about the birth outcome that translates at times into a turning away from the joy at birth. Brenda's contribution to the gathering is to ensure a positive outcome and safeguard the potential for joy to irrupt and open possibilities to all there. Working as a team and being there in the right way to achieve the best outcome contributes to joy at birth awakening.

Sometimes this is about leaping in to do something; sometimes a leaping ahead mode of care is appropriate to ensure space for the other to find their own possibilities going forward. For Brenda leaping in professionally at birth may ensure that leaping ahead into future parenthood is even possible. The shared mood at birth shows how participants can turn towards and attune to joy at birth or not. There seems to be a fine line between leaping-in excessively that can potentially cover up the joyful experience and leaping-ahead that gives freedom to joy's expression in the gathering. Yet neither situation is static. Sometimes standing back or jumping in and intervening are necessary to safeguard joy's awakening and future possibilities.

There is a shared experience at birth that brings people together, connects others and gathers. To be in the world of birth is Being-with-others. Being-with-others at birth discloses how participants are intimately concerned with each other in a connected way and how such gathering at birth matters even if coming from different points of view and responsibilities.

Mood as contagious

It can be difficult for the special mood around birth to be protected. When others at birth do not attune into the collective joy and turn away, something alters in the atmosphere. Simone [midwife] describes this:

> The longer I'm a midwife I feel that feeling is sometimes just there at birth. It is just an inner calmness that probably transmits because if you have tension, then it can spread. I think that if there's somebody who is tense, even a furrowed brow or an anxious expression, everybody is very aware of what's happening. If there was tension, if there's concern, then it radiates out changing the feeling in the room.

There is a sense of mood as contagious. An individual may not share the collective mood, failing to attune to the atmosphere of the moment. Such individuals may resist collective mood and discord can mount as seen in previous chapter when disturbance and disruption by others was revealed. Simone reveals how someone can enter the birth space and change the atmosphere. It appears joy at birth is vulnerable to being covered over due to the contagious nature of other powerful ways of attuning such as fear and anxiety. Fear can hold potential to bury and deny access to joy's awakening at birth. Yet, equally, an unknown person can enter the birth space and be at once synchronised with the joy, resulting in a harmonic shared communication.

Simone tells of how an inner calm can be transmitted that safeguards joy. It seems that joy's potency at birth can radiate out and overwhelm but the possibility for turning away from joy is always there. Even when joy is not experienced due to tiredness or feeling uninspired, birth is no less special. We need to allow joy to arrive and interact with us. Heidegger (1995:82) tells us that a mood can "approach us and tell us what it wants, what is going on with it". To deny this would be to remain uncompleted in what could have been revealed to us at birth in that moment when joy arrives. Seemingly, to be in the birth gathering in the 'right way' is an art.

As mentioned previously, it is important to acknowledge that birth does not always unfold positively due to adverse social and medical concerns. Things can and do go wrong at birth and not all attune to joy at birth for myriad reasons. In these circumstances the potential for joy at birth remains quiescent. The previous chapter spoke of a maternal death and my own experience working with stillbirth. Here I remember a challenging social situation when a baby is born for adoption:

> The mother did not want to look at the baby as it was taken, I felt so sad and wanted the mother so much to just look at what she had created thinking that it would heal her pain. The hospital staff wanted to be near and hold the baby. The baby was still a miracle even though unwanted. That just made it feel all the sadder.

(Reflective diary)

There is something about birth that aligns us with each other and with what birth 'is'. I felt sad as the joy at birth was not allowed to be awakened around the birth of this baby being placed for adoption. This left sadness in its wake. Yet we gathered around the birth, the mother there in her silent pain, the hospital staff drawing near with concern. This was a privative experience leaving a deep feeling of un-rightness. I remember feeling near and connected to the vulnerable baby and to the staff on the labour ward in a more profound way than before.

Disharmony and resonance

Birth is essentially a 'we-world', a world gathered into belongingness and togetherness. The occasion of birth however it unfolds is always with-other and attuned collectively. When this is fractured there is unease. Birth can harbour co-existing joys and sorrows; it can be celebrated, tragic, or not wanted yet para-doxically always gathers us near. Something surprisingly ineffable coalesces into precious uniting wholeness even when challenges arise. John [father] illustrates how these challenges are not to be understood as bad:

> Birth is a good challenge. It was an opportunity for us to grow closer together. It was exciting, lots of unknowns which added to the excitement and opened up lots of possibilities.

The birth was an exciting challenge for John. There were many unknowns as the planned 'natural birth' transformed into a long induction of labour for post-maturity and epidural analgesia. Yet the events leading to the birth seemed to intensify the meeting of their newborn and the irrupting of joy and love that surrounded that moment. Sometimes it is not events but those present at births that are the chal-lenge as they lack resonance with others in the gathering, although this is not always the case. Here Steve [obstetrician] eloquently describes how birth holds power to heal misaligned others by assailing them in joy when they come near:

> Whoever is there as the baby's birth including me, gets realigned with their own sense of the occasion. Initially I and others may have not been quite taken on how significant it was and then when we realise how it's affecting everyone around you, I realise how it is still a big deal. Sometimes I can be pleasantly surprised by the impact birth has on a bloke who is otherwise very gruff and staunch who is overwhelmed by the baby and completely taken with the whole thing in ways I hadn't expected.

Others can, by their affective moods, infect the situation beforehand but birth itself seems to override these. Discord can be removed in an instant due to joy's contagious nature as expressions of joy become sketched on the gathered faces. Others bring their mood and join and merge into the symphony as the orchestra tunes in as one. Birth seemingly like the conductor of an orchestra attunes the gathering at birth into forgiving any previous disharmony. Even grumpy, stoic personalities are affected by joy's forgiving transformative power as it spreads through the gathering. Tui narrates how others previously in discord are gathered together as joy invokes forgiveness:

> I didn't trust my daughter's friend. I had all these strange feelings towards her. I felt that she was intruding. But then I loved her, happy for her to be in the room and thought she was wonderful. I gave her a big hug immediately after the birth. The moment that my grandson came out, everybody was just wonderful. I loved everyone – even the midwife that rushed everything.

Tui speaks of a sudden change in relationships, how those previously in discord become aligned. The suddenness and overwhelming dynamic nature of birth can strike at the soul of participants who may until that point be engrossed in professional or family concerns. There is a shared sentiment that beckons tenderness, a sense of accord that seems to erase any discord. Amy [mother] finds that a congenial way of being is initiated at birth opening possibilities for forgiveness and drawing others nearer than were previously:

> The doctor hurt me more than anyone else, but then my daughter was suddenly there and there was so much love.

Amy attunes joyfully following a traumatic forceps birth. She can traverse the challenges of labour cultivating instant magnanimity following the birth that draws the doctor nearer. Joy is revealed as having the power to unite and forgive.

Gathering responsibility

Whatever the perspectives there is a feeling of responsibility to be close to birth to assist and help even if at times those called do not want to be there or attune asynchronously with the rest of the gathering. This sense of responsibility calls participants to attend and provide care as birth approaches. For family, friends, and health care professionals this beckoning responsibility can be demanding. Tui reflects on how she gathers at birth with a feeling of joyous responsibility:

> I'm reminded in the baby that I'm holding, about both the joy of life and also the kind of fragility of life, knowing that I hold life and death in my hands. I have this precious baby, but it's up to me to sustain this life, and make sure that she's alright. And that she's alive. There is the joy of a responsibility. There's nothing that ever touches that.

Tui is confronted with life and possible death simultaneously. The precariousness of life and death juxtaposed at birth intensifies the experience.

To be called to birth may not always feel joyous. The responsibility to attend may be experienced as mundane despite its significance. Obstetricians and midwives are constantly exposed to the phenomenon of birth in its many guises. They have professional responsibilities which they are called to attend. Does continual exposure to birth lesson the significance of being part of the gathering at birth? Steve [senior obstetrician] speaks of how birth can become a routinised mundane job:

> I can sometimes lose sight of that specialness, because I've been involved with lots and sometimes it does get routine. It's always hard to be too excited at 3 o'clock in the morning, exhilarated by it all, but on the whole I think there is an element of ... (silent), while it is part of my job; it can become more of a routine in most cases (silent pause). Sometimes I'm there in the exhilaration of complex births and it can be very intense, but it also can be, to coin a phrase, 'bog standard', woman comes and pushes out baby, that's probably less exhilarating because I have less at stake. But on the other hand, it's still a very significant and special even when it's not so exhilarating. I am not so cold hearted to regard some births as, 'just another'; when I get to that I'll retire.

Although Steve derives satisfaction from the times in which his specialist skills are called upon, he finds it challenging to always attune to birth as special. The joy at birth can become taken-for-granted, so familiar that it fades into the background. Steve relates how he is *"thinking probably a couple deliveries blurring into one"*. However, he is reminded that all births are significant and special. He calls himself back to that appreciation that 'something' lies in the background of all births and says that it would be time to retire when he loses that connection. Not to be able to acknowledge the significance and specialness of birth he claims would be a *"sign of cold heartedness"*.

Being-there at birth is always significant even if buried under workloads, routines, and tiredness. The notion of birth as mundane and "bog standard" arises in the experience of birth when health care providers are there at one birth after another. In such busyness the average, everyday experience of following routines and protocols would appear to dominate birth experiences. Yet participants speak of aligning themselves to the significance of birth despite this, they catch themselves sliding into a tedious everydayness and re-attune to joy in each unique birth experience. Marie [midwife] attempts to hold onto the significance of birth when she is tired:

> For me it is never mundane, each birth is special, and I absolutely do hold onto that. I try without any conscious artificiality to imbue that, I try to be gentle, include the dad, it is their baby. It is not mundane like *'Oh well got a birth, yea, just got two more for the month'*; It is something more special than that. More special than just going out to do a job. I must admit when they ring me at 9 at night to say they are revving up I am finding it harder to be excited [laughs], I think that is why it is time for me to give up. The fact that I am going to be called later in the night is not so exciting to me now. But once I am there, I will put my heart and soul into it.

Being called in the middle of the night can be arduous but once there in the gathering Marie engages fully with her responsibilities. She safeguards the significance of birth despite her feelings because it is always special. Dianne [midwife] has the same approach:

> I can be tired, but I cannot go to that birth with feelings of resentment as I am lucky to be involved with them.

I am reminded how busy hospital birthing units can be stretched by shortages of staff, and of my own self-employed practice when having a busy month with many births expected. In such busy circumstances being there with others at birth is not always so wonderful and joyful. The participants speak about how childbirth professionals contain this tension in their working lives. How would joy at birth be kept awake with such tension? Despite occasional difficulties birth is never mundane and all participants appreciate that being part of the gathering at birth is a privilege.

Privileged gathering

Participants spoke of the privilege of Being-there at birth with-others. Midwives and obstetricians mentioned the uplifting and full-filling quality of their work. They speak of the privileged roles they have that allow access into the intimate lives of others at special and vulnerable moments:

> I felt in awe and just so privileged to be there but not interrupt it, but to be present and give them what they wanted and just facilitate their ability to do that. To be at birth is very fulfilling.
>
> (Simone – midwife)

> To be part of and involved in birth is very privileged. They don't have that emotional relationship with me nor me with them if we haven't met before, but none the less, I am present at the birth of their baby; an event which is special to them and which is special to me as well. It's a special privilege being part of someone's life and being able to either help it or make it better or intervene to make the final outcome the best it can be.
>
> (Carol – senior obstetrician)

The intimacy and specialness of a baby being born is unique. Steve [obstetrician] is drawn to his work as he is exposed to life's possibility: *"I enjoy working at the right end of life with the demographic I work with"*. Health care professionals have unique roles at birth. The obstetricians and midwives in this study care about their work because of its significance. They gather in the world of birth, meet themselves there with others, and at once become who they are with-others. They feel honoured, privileged, and enjoy being there in the birth gathering doing what they can to assist in new life arriving.

Birth acts as a mobilisation of others into action which highlights the responsibility inherent in gathering at birth, to be at birth is a sharing of a social horizon in which they all 'touch' each other. Professional maternity care providers, birthing women, and birth partners are touched and drawn into the gathering. Health care professionals are similarly affected despite their roles and responsibilities. Participants, including obstetricians, describe a magical feeling full of awe and peace as they gather in their various roles at birth.

To be there at birth is to care. For Heidegger, Dasein's fundamental way of Being-in-the-world is care. This is not care for particular things but care as our fundamental comportment to the world. Participants find themselves thrown into the world of birth in a concerning way dealing with what matters most to them. This desire to care and actualise concerns into actions is an aspect of Being-with at birth that contributes to the birth gathering. Participants tell of how they are beckoned to gather at birth and intuit the need to act responsibly. Families and friends draw near out of responsibility to care about something significant. Midwives and obstetricians too draw near out of professional responsibility with their own set of concerns.

As those at birth gather around in their various roles, I wondered to whom the gathering belongs; whose joy is being safeguarded? Health care professionals are there but seemingly in some sense not there. They are often not intimate or significant others for the birthing family, yet they are part of the gathering around birth. For example, Marie [midwife] explains how she tries to be there amongst the unfolding intimacy and remain unnoticed:

> She had this very gentle birth. The student was delighted to see the big bulging bag of fore waters in front of the baby's head. The baby was born in the caul[1]. It is funny it's not me experiencing this; it is part of something else. It is like I stand back a little bit because it is their baby. I just want them to welcome their baby and I am just the pair of gloves; I am trying to protect their first moment with their baby. There is a joy seen in their eyes as they see their baby for the 1st time. Apart from drying the baby as we have to do [laughs] and addressing safety things I tend to sit back a bit.

Marie's experience of birth does not derive from her appropriation of the gathering joy for herself, yet she is there amidst and part of the shared experience. Marie experiences a joy that is both personal and impersonal that awakens once the baby has arrived safely. Marie is able to stand back and be the '*pair of gloves*'. Her role as midwife is not to take over the joy or be an overtly visible member of the gathering. She acknowledges how significant birth is to the family and does not want to get in the way of their joyous gathering. Yet she is more than a pair of gloves.

Marie mirrors joy in her embodied expressions, actions, silences, and language moving through the spaces of birth sensitively. Paradoxically she witnesses the birth and, in that moment, attunes joyfully as part of the gathering even as she attempts to remain invisible. The joy is *who she is* as she *meets herself* in that intimate moment. In her safeguarding of joy, she provides a space for joy to be awakened. This is truly an artful way to practice and an example of leaping ahead in her care.

There is a mutual gifting of joy within the birth gathering. A reciprocal joy that brings all into increasing nearness to one another at birth. A special nearness that is awakened by joy that invites all into the gathering beyond the confines of professional roles, apparent tensions and any discord.

Significance of relationships

The strength of others gathers at birth in a seemingly reciprocal manner as relationships are revealed as central to joy's awakening. Whether relationships are formed prior to birth or not are essential to joys awakening is unclear. Dianne [midwife] alludes to previously formed relationships facilitating something more:

> If I'm doing a duty at the hospital and this woman comes in off the street, I try my hardest to connect with her, I've got to keep the relationship intact during that birth, even though I may be pushed and stretched and be really challenged. But I would be letting myself down if I didn't try because at the end of the day, she's having a baby and I do still get excited, but the joy is much more with somebody I know.

This is an illustration of how joy at birth can be shared and deepened in the process of relationship building. This is a celebration of the partnership and continuity of care models of midwifery care. Providing care seems easier with someone known prior to birth. Yet Dianne still gets excited and attunes joyfully even when she does not know the family beforehand as birth is always a significant event; although new relationships demand more effort on her part. The feeling of joy, however, seems deepened and more accessible when Dianne gets to know families before birth. Conversely, Carol [obstetrician] describes how working in the public hospitals rarely provides opportunity to have a prior relationship:

> I don't know the women I don't have that relationship with them. So, it is a much more clinical; someone calls me, I need to assess the situation, I need to make a recommendation and get the baby delivered. It's much more clinical and the emotional part of it for me about being excited or happy or satisfied about a birth, that's much less now, it's changed. It was that relationship part of it that was important for me to feel much more emotionally involved in births. Whereas now I would say it's much more clinical; it's my job to get this baby delivered and as safely as possible. Sometimes I feel sad about that sometimes not. I mean it's easier emotionally to just walk in, get my job done and go. But I miss that emotional part of it too when you have much more invested in these women's lives.

Carol reveals loss regarding the reciprocal relationships that she had with her patients in private practice. She reminisces about how she was able to be attuned with the family and experience joy more readily. She describes how her job has become far more clinical since working in the public sector. Reciprocal relationships are important to Carol. She misses the bonding afforded by the relationship and how that engenders connectedness and being more touched by joy at birth.

Being-with-other in prior relationship is an issue in Dianne and Carol's stories for the joy to be fully awakened. The notion of relational continuity has been shown to be central to positive birth experiences for women and midwives (e.g. Homer *et al.*, 2019; Dahlberg and Aune, 2013; Sandall *et al.*, 2016; Downe *et al.*, 2016). Perhaps pre-formed relationships help safeguard joy so that it awakens and presences more intensely when the baby is born. However, Steve [obstetrician] states that an already-there relationship is not essential to this experience of joy of birth:

> If I am seeing somebody for the 1st time in labour I have to provide some assistance that's perhaps equally as satisfying. To know that I can actually reassure them and give them the confidence to do what they need to do, even when I don't have the lead up of knowing them for weeks and weeks. So that's one aspect of the public practice that I quite enjoy.

Although Steve distinguishes between private and public practice, he recognises that they both hold something for him. In private practice he can build a rapport with patients before the birth whereas in public work he is often called in to assist the birth with no prior knowing. He enjoys the familiarity of private work but also the need to develop a quick rapport in public work is satisfying. His story uncovers how joy as an aspect of being-with others at birth appears to awaken regardless of prior relationships. I have had similar personal experiences during locum work:

> She was pushing on all fours, I had not met her, only heard her say '*come its now coming!*' on the phone 20 minutes before. Shortly after I arrived the baby was born, she looked up and we smiled, we saw each other for the first time, we had never met before. There was such overwhelming joy in the room I was so thrilled to be there.
>
> (Reflective diary)

Prior professional relationships with women can potentially augment the intensity of joy at birth allowing joy to awaken at birth more easily. Moreover, the notion of needing familiarity with each other at birth in order to attune joy-fully at birth has not been explicitly revealed in the data. This may point to the affirming experiences that core midwifery [non case-loading hospital-based midwives] enjoy.

This inquiry suggests that even when there are no prior relationships participants can be overwhelmed by the joy at birth if they choose to turn towards it. Being-there connected with-others at birth with or without prior relationship is revealed as special in and of itself. The importance and significance of relationships creating an affirming atmosphere at birth has been previously explored (Berg *et al.*, 2012) and relationships built over time have been shown to contribute to safe rural practice (Crowther and Smythe, 2016). Yet pre-formed relationships have not been revealed as being the sole determining factor for the mood of joy at birth to awaken.

What is apparent is that all are called into nearness when a baby is born. Seemingly the closer the actual birth the nearer others appear to gather. In this gathering 'others' are not meant to signify *everyone else*, but rather all others of whom *all individuals* are part: "The world is always the one that I share with Others. The world of Dasein is a with-world. Being-in is Being-with-Others. Their Being-in-themselves within-the-world is Dasein-with" (Heidegger, 1927/1962: 155). Being-with is an existential characteristic of Dasein, part of its structure; that is to say, 'Being-in-the-world' is 'Being-with-others'. Essentially 'Being-with-others-in-the-world-of-birth' is an inseparable unified phenomenon. It is a facticity (e.g. quality, condition, or attribute) of our existence.

Participant roles, cultural expectations, and history coalesce into a relational web of significance as shared joyous gathering. 'Being-with-others-within-the-world-of-birth' is inseparable from the shared lived-experience of joy at birth. To connect the previous sentence together with hyphens is an attempt to foreground an interconnected totality that is birth. Participants are confronted with the majesty of a continuum of life begetting life that reminds them of their interconnectedness with others. There seems to be a gathering strength and joyful anticipation that provokes a welcomed submission to the world-of-birth which affords a glimpse of unknown possibilities. Participants are at the mercy of the world-of birth, because that is their facticity from which we cannot escape "Dasein, in so far as it is, has submitted itself already to a world which it encounters, and this submission belongs to its Being" (Heidegger, 1927/1962: 121).

The sudden moment of birth appears to attune participants joyfully. A joy that suspends and resolves worldly concerns, preferences, distractions, and gifts the possibility to transcend the voice of the One (even if only for a short while). As they submit to the clemency afforded by joy at birth, they find themselves surprised and gathered in an unexpected experience beyond words and are called from mediocrity:

> When I see the baby is actually coming the protocols and procedures are not so evident anymore; then it is the wonder and the joy.
>
> (Marie – midwife)

There is a sense that Marie is called to do what she does from a silent call of conscience. What is revealed is a spirit of generosity and compassion in this silent call to care. As she gathers with others at birth, she is no longer tethered by everyday banality of being dissolved in the One. She ceases to be an adherent to the dictates of the One, finding herself freer and not totally fallen into the levelling effect of the One. Attuned joyfully she finds herself authentically with-others, unfettered, unbound, and seeing freely. For a moment Marie is awarded a vision of interconnectedness gifted by joy's arrival.

Being-with-others at birth is sacred

The moment of joy at birth points to something profound that touches those present. The relational quality is constitutive of Being-with at birth and is significant. Those that gather at birth attune to 'something' human, shared, and precious which they appear to safeguard. This joyous gathering speaks of unity, protection, fellowship; a bringing and joining together within a shared abode. There is a gathering and sense of belonging, dwelling, and homecoming. Birth joy seemingly brings the possibility of wholeness in our lives that is beyond secular and mundane interpretations.

The gathering at birth is more than ensuring safety and survival of mother and baby. Perhaps the gathering is something sacred wherever and however that may be understood. Even within medicalised environments participants speak of sheltering something precious at birth as they gather near and attune joyfully when a baby arrives. They safeguard joy's awakening so that its light can illuminate the way beyond everydayness. Bartlett (2001) warned us at the turn of the twenty-first century that emphasising "safety" over "sacred" would reduce the experience of birth to something secular. Birth as sacred is hard to articulate and points to both something and nothing. But this 'nothing' hints at something unrevealed. As Rudolf Otto (1917/1923) tells us in his germinal work, *The Idea of the Holy*, nothing is always in contrast to something:

> By this 'nothing' is meant not only that of which nothing can be predicated, but that which is absolutely and intrinsically other than and opposite of everything that is and can be thought.
>
> (29)

Perhaps we need to heed Bartlett's warning lest we cover over something of significance when we gather at birth.

Conclusion

The moment of joy at birth is revealed as a collectively experienced blessing beyond everyday concerns and our capacity to understand. Seemingly joy beckons and gathers those there at birth gifting the possibility to 'see', 'meet', and 'connect' with each other anew. The phenomenon joy at birth is revealed as joyous gathering, a joy that unfolds through the childbirth year often co-existing with potential fears and anxieties until its full awakening at the actual birth that gathers others near into a shared abode. The notion of gathering at birth uncovers a glimpse of something extraordinarily quintessential that lies in the background familiarity of birth, reminding us of our being-with-others is to be in the world. At significant 'once in a lifetime events' such as birth the with-ness of others stands out more pressingly as important to us. Yet this gathering at birth points to something more than merely Being-with-others and more than physical bodies coming together in a physical location concerned with safety and bio-medical outcomes. It is a moment of profound significance that draws us near into relational gathering, it is something *we* feel individually and collectively countenancing the sacred to awaken and emerge in our lives.

Birth calls us to joyous gathering

> Life births in anxious anticipation
> in silent calling
> Between;
> darkness light
> calm noise
> loud quiet
> A struggling flower shooting upwards
> through the ancestral sod,
> desires the warmth of sun – relief!
> Glorious expansion to connecting sky,
> reaching up opening to joy
> sun-kissed in a passionate embrace as
> roots burrow down into ancient depths
> holding and secure, tangled with others before
> She reaches up into pristine newness,
> petals unfurl yearningly
> Such fragrance, such joy, such belonging!
> Calling out –
>   Touches,
>   gathers,
>   reveals

Note

1 Being born in the caul is when the baby is born whilst in its intact amniotic sac. The sac of fluids only ruptures open after the birth of the baby.

References

Bartlett, W.D. (2001). Building sacred traditions in birth. *Midwifery Today with International Midwife*, 24.

Berg, M., Ólafsdóttir, O.A., and Lundgren, I. (2012). A midwifery model of woman-centred childbirth care – In Swedish and Icelandic settings. *Sexual and Reproductive Healthcare*, 3, pp. 79–87.

Crowther, S. and Smythe, E. (2016). Open, trusting relationships underpin safety in rural maternity a hermeneutic phenomenology study. *BMC Pregnancy Childbirth*, 16, p. 370.

Dahlberg, U. and Aune, I. (2013). The woman's birth experience: The effect of interpersonal relationships and continuity of care. *Midwifery*, 29(4), pp. 407–415.

Downe, S., Finlayson, K., Tuncalp, Ö., and Metin Gülmezoglu, A. (2016). What matters to women: A systematic scoping review to identify the processes and outcomes of antenatal care provision that are important to healthy pregnant women. *BJOG: An International Journal of Obstetrics & Gynaecology*, 123, pp. 529–539.

Heidegger, M. (1927/1962). *Being and Time*. New York: Harper.

Heidegger, M. (1995). *The Fundamental Concepts of Metaphysics: World, Finitude, Solitude*. Bloomington, IN: Indiana University Press.

Homer, C., Brodie, P., Sandall, J., and Leap, N. (2019). *Midwifery Continuity of Care: A Practical Guide*. London: Elsevier.

Merewether, J. (2013). *Heart and Hands – A History of the Struggle to Protect Healthy Childbirth in Australia*. Australia: Go Girl Productions, 75 mins.

Otto, R. (1917/1923). *The Idea of the Holy (Das Heilige)*. London: Oxford University Press.

Sandall, J., Soltani, H., Gates, S., Shennan, A., and Devane, D. (2016). Midwife-led continuity models versus other models of care for childbearing women. *Cochrane Database of Systematic Reviews*, 4, n.p.

Wojtkowiak, J. and Crowther, S. (2018). An existential and spiritual discussion about childbirth: Contrasting spirituality at the beginning and end of life. *Spirituality in Clinical Practice*, 5, pp. 261–272.

7 Joy as temporal mystery

The previous chapters uncovered joy as embodied, spatial joy, and joy as a gathering quality at birth. What began to surface was a special felt-time. A quality of felt-time – or temporal experience – which uncovered aesthetic and mysterious qualities of space and silences that attune into deeper contemplation. Birth was revealed as unfolding within an extraordinary moment that included the experience of unseen others, the feeling that holy-others draw near; others that are so near as to be unnoticed and others that bring comfort. In such a felt-time new insights and deepening sense of connection unfolded.

How to name that which is ineffable and mysterious?

Joy at birth is made up of many threads that hold the tapestry of the lived-experience together as a gathering whole that appears temporal and mysterious. Although birth is part of everyday life, it confounds our ability to comprehend its gathering wholeness. To come face to face with joy confronts us with a mystery that is more than everydayness and the ability to comprehend an experience "which in our brief lives we can hardly make a start of fathoming" (Gray, 1970: 229). The mystery at birth remains ineffable, beyond words, unfolding within a sense of time and others that are more timeless and spacious than words alone can convey. This mystery is difficult to 'say' but is at the same time something so simple and so near within the experiences of participants awaiting expression.

Splendour of the simple[1]

To stay within the splendour of the simple is to appreciate the ineffability of languaging that 'something' is experienced at birth. In other words, by remaining close to the thing itself and keeping it simple, we begin to reveal what has always in some way always been there beyond our ability to articulate yet within the lived experience itself. Hermeneutic phenomenology teaches us that nothing is totally revealed nor fully concealed – it is always both. Joy at birth dwells in between spaces, within a liminal place and is part of who we are and between who we are. It is bursting with possibilities that are always surfacing if we were to look closely.

To look closely requires we open ourselves to that which is simple and always there. This is about coming to birth, not as controllers speaking to the experience, neither is this about measuring and capturing a finite absolute truth. It is calling us to be open to the possibilities unfolding at birth which speak to us in each moment. Appreciating the simple about birth requires thinking beyond traditions so that new insights can surface. Birth has become so complex, surrounded by facts and things to do that the simplicity of how birth affects us alludes. The overly analytic approach can serve to close down the possibility to enter into new understandings out of defined fields of knowledge. Prior knowing can be problematic but has been shown to be always there. The truth of birth in its simplest terms often remains hidden, even forgotten. The origin is what lies deeply behind all beginnings of thought and conceptualisation. This is therefore not the historical, cultural, and bio-medical understandings of birth but the simple taken-for-granted reality of what lies hidden in the experience of being at the birth of a baby.

To focus on the splendour of the simple illuminates what is already there yet hidden. The simple is not immediately accessible or evident; it requires sustained contemplative thought. This is a persistent staying close to the experience, enabling whatever wants to show itself to be seen. The splendour of the simple is a call to return to what finds us gathered together in a new freedom where truth begins to be revealed. To think about joy at birth simply is to penetrate what is going on; what it is showing itself to be. The simple is always just out of reach, just out of sight and hearing yet always somehow there. Burrowing deep into the wonder of birth is to attune to joy and arrive at the splendour of the simple that awaits our embrace; however, we may feel, or not feel, at birth there is always the potential to open ourselves to new horizons of understanding.

The simple gestures to our always already interconnectedness with what are known and unknown. Splendour of simplicity is the call to see the phenomenon from within, not as dispassionate observer, and requires stillness, space, and silence.

This is a call for 'feeling' the words as they speak the unsayable; bringing presence to what is hidden:

> Of presence. I say well-hidden because, as you might realise by now, in many places silence is key, and these things are rarely talked about.
>
> (Rethmann, 2006: 52)

Heidegger (1971/2001) argues that genuine thinking on a phenomenon is poetic. This is not necessarily in verse form but in the use of language which provides space and silence for something more to arise. Lauren Hunter in her hermeneutic phenomenological study on midwives' knowing in childbirth contends that poems help to "capture a unique and fresh aspect about lived-experience..." (Hunter, 2008: 406). Poetic prose allows a way of revealing more about the time of birth which is felt and how such experience is significant and meaningful. The poetic form, according to Lauren, is "a way of putting non-scientific ways of knowing onto paper" (ibid.: 406). Poetry is thus the "saying of the unconcealment of what is" (Heidegger, 1971/2001: 74), a form of expression that brings "the unsayable as such into a world" (ibid.: 74).

The simplicity of words in poetic form provides access to more aesthetic knowing about birth not normally captured in academic text. The poetic form helps bring joy at birth to something felt which allows its truth to surface and be brought to presence in the silences and spaces of feelings and contemplative thinking. As Rethman (2006) adds, "… instead of allowing the silence to melt into language, a device to propel a plot, it should be perhaps left as what it is: a connection with something larger than the self" (46). As Carol McDonald (2007) claims poetic language does not describe or explain but whispers meaning to us creating an experience for the reader. Joy at birth requires space and silence to be felt and heard. Spaces and silences are able to presence joy's simplicity, inviting you the reader to come from the shadows of your forest paths into the clearing and hear the whispers.

Over the remaining pages of this chapter I suspend traditional prose and scholarly ways of thinking and reading which may obscure the path into the clearing. Emerging from participant experiences poems, using their words, are crafted. Each poem ends with an essence forming a final poem (see page 160) that glimpses qualities and hints at meaning surfaced from the temporal lived-experience of the phenomenon. I invite you to immerse yourself in the splendour of the simple and allow the whispers of meaning to create an experience as you read through the stories and poems that follow.

No laboratory can cook this up!

The second baby was delivered in its gestational sack still swimming around with its hair floating like a little mermaid and its hands bouncing against the sack. The baby kind of splattered out and started breathing. The Dad looked over and instantly within seeing burst into tears and then the mother burst into tears out of relief and joy. That was quite a strong experience, it felt like seeing creation. It felt like something out of this world! Seeing that baby surviving in a sack and in an instant changing to being an independent little human being was amazing. I don't know exactly what happened in that moment of birth. Even though I am medical, and my primary goal was to act as a medical person to facilitate the birth I can't remove myself from those beautiful experiences and enjoying it. It is more than the medical stuff to me it's spiritual.

There's no laboratory you could cook that up in! It really seemed like it was just all being knitted up together. Knowing that each and every one is knitted together in that same manner. It's a miracle. If it were all just chance and atoms that happened to fall together in the right configuration it probably wouldn't be so impressive. It's the gesture or the action that shows us that there is continuity, there's more purpose to life. The process carries on the same as it has done for thousands of years. The fact that it keeps happening with such continuity is a good symbol to us to keep hoping for better things. Birth is a symbol of the continuity of life and gives us value for our lives, giving birth value.

(Brenda – obstetrician)

Seeing the baby
tears burst out
Being touched
simply amazing

Being in a strong experience
being witness to miracles
Seeing creation unfold
all knitted together
No laboratory can cook this up!

We are created beings part of creation
being-in the continuity of life
Birth is spiritual
gifting value and purpose to life

Birth is something out of this world

What happens at birth is something out of this world...

Instinctive embedded knowing

The baby came and there was a little bit of a breath and then straight up to mum, and then baby cried and everybody is elated. The joy, the atmosphere changes [click of fingers] just like that. There was lots of tension and then it shifted to joy, relief, release and celebration. There is an interaction with something and sense of being full. Birth exposes me to something else that doesn't happen every day. It's an instinctive, embedded knowing; a momentous event generation after generation of women having birthed that doesn't change. The repetition and connection is all part of the significance of it; a link to the thing. The pool of the universe, the ocean of souls.

(Simone – midwife)

Joy arrives just like that!
It's a celebration
all are elated

Being exposed to something other
Being at a momentous event
not an everyday experience

Feeling and being full
feeling the continuum
feeling connection to the thing –
the universe,
the pool of souls

Deep knowing

... drawing forth a deep knowing ...

Right there in that moment

The past, present and future are right there, in that moment. That moment of birth is when your ancestors are here now and your future yet to come is right there in that moment of birth. Then they take their breath, it's that essence – just the moment of a baby being born, it's like the essence of everything meeting. Birth is not just a medical event or a purely biological event. I don't believe and feel that it's solely up to us there is the mystical going on definitely. That's not always what I feel in that moment, but it's that feeling that keeps me true to why I became a midwife.

(Anahera – midwife)

Being at past, present and future
essence of 1st breath
essence of all meeting

Being 'right there' in that moment
Ancestors 'right there' in that moment
Inheritors 'right there' in that moment

Not just bio-medical
something not in our control

Feeling something mystical
that keeps me true to Being myself

*... a mystical feeling right there in that moment
bringing me to myself ...*

Sacred moment of ending and beginning

It was like a powerful moment that is somehow sacred. I think it was kind of what he was doing that made it powerful and sacred. The sacredness was coming from him, he was controlling everything. You could only go along with it and surrender to what he has to do. There were no concerns, birth was conclusion to a long anticipation; the three of us having achieved the amazing thing. Having him on me at the end was something altogether different. Birth was the end and this is the beginning. They're not one and the same.

(Cathy – mother)

Being in a powerful moment
sacralised moment

Being surrendered to that moment
everything coming from my baby
he controlled all
being in his flow

We become family
Birth is the end
is the beginning

*... a moment of ending and beginning
calling to us to surrender ...*

Timeless joy

There is a great sense of joy and laughter. It was very timeless, that was part of the mood. It was a timeless preciousness that touched me to my core that I will not get back; it's never going to happen again.

(Amy – mother)

Being in joy and laughter
being in timeless joy
being in timeless preciousness

Deeply touched
never to come again

... a unique moment of timeless joy that deeply touches ...

Ancestral connections

I caught my grandchild; I had this face in front of me that wasn't a face, that just kind of morphed through some faces that I recognise so rapidly that it was like jelly almost forming into a face that I knew – of my grand-parents and my father and heaps of faces that I didn't know until it came to her face. It eventually settled with her face. I was watching, thinking, 'Oh! What is this? What's going on?' It was the most Amazing thing. I've got no idea how long it took before she settled into whom she is, but the faces of all her ancestors on both sides were there. Just for fractions of a second until it settled into her face.

I think part of what's building is that each of those people brings their own past and their own ancestors into that moment, so you've got this con-centration, you've got this massive crowd of thousands in this room and all that energy is focused on this little being. It's almost as if that call also comes from the baby. The baby calls and focuses this massive love and energy and joy. But it's not just a one-way thing. The crowd of thousands that have arrived are also calling out. It comes from these generations and generations and generations that have gone before. It is almost like a folding in and out of past and future.

In that moment past and future collide. I'm very aware of all of my ancestors being there. I'm also aware this baby is our future in this little tiny being, that's struggling to breathe – this is our future, this is an amazing feeling– as everything comes together in that moment. There is a kind of spiritual fullness, like being in gentleness. All of the past, all of the stuff that's gone into making me, and all of the stuff that's coming out of me is There! Right there! Like a potential. All is how it should be.

(Tui – grandmother)

Being in amazement
with mystery
awed
feeling full

Being-with those that have come before
The stuff that made me now comes through me
Timeless moment –
right there right now
Everything comes together

Past, present and future collide
folding one into the other
Baby calls out
others call out

Cast of thousands arrive
love energy joy awakens
from the past
possibility potential hope welcomed

All is alright -
this is being alive!

... a felt moment that all is how it should be

Being-with those that came before and Being-with those that are to come ...

Numinous experience and gratitude

There were waves of tears as he came. The soft tears were thankfulness and gratitude to God, to the universe and life for producing the moment. The moment is the miracle, this whole human being coming into the world; it is a miracle of the universe to produce my son. There is a definite sense of awe in that moment; an awestruck type of momentousness. The birth of our baby is a cosmic event. Every moment is a cosmic event really but you just get so used to ordinary life that it all starts to seem ordinary. But his birth was so obviously extraordinary that it shocked me out of not seeing everything as miraculous; I was shocked out of my everyday experience and feeling. The birth was so novel, so obviously miraculous that it allowed me to tap into the feeling of wow. Something momentous was happening and I was witnessing and involved with it. Being at the birth last week reminded me that life is actually mystical.

(Karl – father)

Waves of grateful tears
to life, universe,
God

Birth is novel
extraordinary
cosmic

Miraculous moment
Awestruck
shocked from
everydayness

Mystical encounter
Being-with miraculous

... an extraordinary moment of overwhelming gratitude ...

Birth is special

I don't think of birth as an epiphany or a spiritual sacred event or anything like that, it's a part of life; it's a very normal life process that is special, that's all. It is not cosmic to me or spiritual or things like that. It's a normal part of life but one we attribute a lot of specialness too! There is something special going on; though I can't define special.

(Carol – obstetrician)

Birth is
Part of life
Normal life process

The moment at birth
Undefinable specialness

... an undefinable special moment in normal life ...

Being touched by sacredness

I remember being quite sort of moved by this birth. They were probably quite a religious family and so a Māori prayer was said that sort of trig-gered a bit of 'something', I suppose a reinforcement of the significance of it and the sacredness of it all; it certainly showed how special it was for them. I could also see that I was obviously part of it and I was touched. I was pleased to be part of it. I was privileged to be a part of that particular birth knowing that this 'something' wouldn't be repeated readily. Sacred-ness and specialness are not the words I would choose, but the sentiment is probably similar.

(Steve – obstetrician)

> Being moved
> Being touched
> Being privileged
> Being grateful
>
> Being triggered by something
> reinforcing significance
> feeling something
> not repeatable
>
> Feeling '*special*'
> Feeling '*sacred*'
>
> *... unrepeatable moment that reminds us ...*

Birth as sacrament

In that split second it was an expression and sacrament of the present moment. When they met their baby, it was a sacrament to me. Sacrament is a sign of God's presence. God's presence is tied up with that wonder thing. I really felt God's presence there welcoming that baby. Birth is God's invitation to be part of creation, who has invited those there in that moment to be part of the creation of this universe in the form of this baby. Being there is privileged [weeps].

(Marie – midwife)

> In that split second
> creation invites
> feeling wonder
> feeling presence
> being in wonder
>
> Birth as sacrament
> Sign of Holy-other's presence
> feeling God's presence
> being invited into Holy presence
> feeling privileged
>
> *... of the wonder and holy presence of being in creation ...*

Imminence

Spirituality is grounded in the reality of what I saw and felt at his birth. Birth was about being alive, being present, being connected, being loved, feeling love, and that sense of being close to that core, to Mother Earth and her sudden heartbeat. Mother Earth was expressing Herself through my body. I needed to surrender and accept that Mother Nature, God or whoever, had it all under control. The birth was very much about seeing, feeling, hearing, that's what really matters.

(Pat – mother)

> Being present
> loved
> close to the core
> Feeling Mother Earth's sudden heartbeat
> birthing through my body
> Acceptance and surrender
> sensing and feeling everything near
> is what mattered
> Birth was being alive

... that feels connected to what matters most ...

There aren't words but there is the experience

There's a company that arrives at birth. This shift is not coming from the baby. Not coming from me or the mother, it's something arriving. A company of spirits that do something magic at that moment providing this joy, this being in love with everyone. It's instantaneous at that moment when the baby comes out. It's a total shift. And everything's ok, people there and the place it is happening it doesn't seem to matter where we are. Ultimately it doesn't matter. I became aware that there was something there and something happening that wasn't of this world. At the same time it is touchable and tangible. This company comes in and stirs up this happiness because I was just totally overcome with it – it's an energy thing. I don't know what it is. Sometimes there aren't words but there is the experience.

(Tui – grandmother)

> Instant moment
> Something shifts at birth
> Company of spirits arrive
> Being stirred up
> Awakening joy, love, and happiness
>
> Being in love with everyone
> Being totally overcome with it all!
> Not of this world
> Experience beyond words

... an experience that stirs us up beyond words

All secular and sacred arts and sciences conjoin into simple gathering, gesturing to a uniting power that holds all parts together in the preceding stories and poems. The phenomenon of joy at birth speaks its own language, from within and beyond known time, it calls us to surrender to it and be attentive to any part which arrives.

A time comes
When you must give yourself
all away, all away
    (Schumacher, 2012: 29)

Surrendering to the path of the simple brings us to a clearing where all can gather. A clearing which provides an open space for revelation of birth's significance and deeper meaning. Joy at birth appears to gather us authentically, opening new ways of seeing beyond everyday concerns that point us home to warmth and tender togetherness. The clearing opens up possibilities yet unknown or anticipated.

No longer veiled by the forest canopy we enter into this clearing in which everyday judgements, concerns, and worries become suspended as joy shines a light on deeper knowing. Protocols and policies fade as the birth experience fully engages us and simply brings us "there" in attuned joy. History, culture, bio-medical sciences, and professional discourses are the trees that decorate the boundaries of the clearing. They threaten to conceal the truth of birth. Yet they all gather whoever and whatever their beginnings in the clearing. The clearing brings us face to face with the origin of birth's ineffable mystery. Such clearing gathers and shelters "formed in being and comes forth as being" (Gadamer, 2007: 135). It is a gathering which "moving-into-nearness" releases us from any sense of willing to think and do things in certain ways (Heidegger, 1959/1969: 67).

Being there at birth is to dwell within a temporal mystery. A felt-time in which we attune joyfully – a joy that authenticates and opens us to new possibilities. To be authenticated in the phenomenological sense is to be released from the dictates of the One and not fallen into familiar and customary ways of being. This is not about personal validation or confirmation. To be authenticated in that moment is be found in a clearing of our Being. This clearing is freedom to be with-others in new ways.

Note

1 "The splendour of the simple" quoted line from *Poetry, Language, Thought*, Chapter 1: The thinker as poet (Heidegger, 1971/2001: 7) from original German 'Die Pracht des Schlichten'. In: *Aus der Erfahrung des Denkens* (1947).

References

Gadamer, H.G. (2007). *The Gadamer Reader: A Bouquet of Later Writings*. Evanston, IL: Northwestern University Press.
Gray, J.G. (1970). Splendor of the simple. *Philosophy East and West*, 20, pp. 227–240.
Heidegger, M. (1959/1969). *Discourse on Thinking*. New York: HarperCollins.
Heidegger, M. (1971/2001). *Poetry, Language, Thought*. New York: HarperCollins.
Hunter, L.P. (2008). A hermeneutic phenomenological analysis of midwives' ways of knowing during childbirth. *Midwifery*, 24, pp. 405–415.
McDonald, C. (2007). Reaching for mother across difference. In: V. Bergum and J. Zalm, eds, *Motherlife: Studies of Mothering Experience*. Alberta, Canada: Pedagon Publishing, pp. 302–315.
Rethmann, P. (2006). On presence. In: J. Goulet and B.G.M., eds, *Extraordinary Anthropology*. London: University of Nebraska Press, pp. 36–52.
Schumacher, L. (2012). *The Stone I Love*. Ashland, OR: Eagle Eye Press.
Whyte, D. (1997). *The House of Belonging: Poems*. Moorhead, MN Many Rivers Press.

Part III
New horizons

8   Kairos and shared natality

We have seen that there is a special moment at birth that contains embodied, spatial, and relational qualities surfacing within a feeling of special time and hinting at nearness with some mysterious-otherness. The moment at birth as temporal mystery was revealed poetically in the last chapter and disclosed something uniquely special in the silences and spaces between and within words. In doing this work new horizons of understanding foreground something of meaning and existential value. The time of birth has been revealed as a profoundly significant temporal experience that touches us on multiple levels. In this chapter I name this time Kairos time and describe the numinous[1] experiences that Kairos brings to birth.

Although clock time is part of the experience it is the personal, lived, subjective felt-time that is revealed in the experience of being at birth. It is special time that signals a moment of significance beyond everydayness that follows birth, the moment is "transcendent" beyond our individual everyday lives and concerns. There is a sense of disconnection and suspension of time as the tempo of clock time alters. Concerns over clock time dissolve into something without boundaries at birth.

In my own practice, checking the clock for the exact time of birth feels like a consciously imposed professional act which seems so unimportant. Although clock time is required if, and when, a baby or mother needs resuscitation. The first meeting with a new baby is more often a time of hushed calmness. In these moment(s) joy often awaits, awakening at the opportune time and disclosing the gathering of something extraordinary. In that moment a shift occurs wherein previous worries vanish leaving a feeling that all is well. A sense of excitement and awestruck amazement infuses the moment that resonates with concord, empowerment, belongingness, and harmony. Birth unfolds in a felt-time that is sacred, acting as catalyst for change and deeply stirs us. In this deep stirring of the soul a timeless knowing awareness that is not always conscious is able to surface. When we find ourselves at the moment of birth something confronts us in a moment of Kairos time.

Kairos time

Kairos time is qualitative, something beyond chronos time which is measurable and ordered. Kairos is an ancient Greek word that means the right moment or opportune or critical moment (Kazenshe, 2004); a "passing instant when an opening appears which must be driven through with force if success is to be achieved" (White, 1987: 13). Labour and birth can involve overcoming many hurdles requiring extreme effort and surrender to natural forces. Yet from such a moment something new can build upon what is already there.

Box 8.1 Kairos time at birth

- Moment both in time and beyond time
- Inclusive and more than lineal and cyclic/process time
- An intensity of felt-time
- An indeterminate time when tempo of time changes
- Moments that are special, extraordinary, unrepeatable, exceptional
- Time that is astounding, novel, and precious
- Unexpected time that is surprising, sudden, powerful, overwhelming
- Time of amazement and exciting feelings
- Time sacred in nature, spiritual, mysterious with potential for unseen otherness
- Significant and meaningful time
- Gathering, connecting relational quality of time
- Time that brings forth deep knowing and remembrance
- Time that alters current and prior perceptions

Source: adaped from Crowther *et al.*, 2015

In the context of this study, Kairos time is an indeterminate moment of time in which something special and sacred happens (see Box 8.1). It describes a transitional and liminal state outside of time, place, and culture. At birth a feeling of journeying into the future is revealed from unknown and known pasts. There is a sense of emergent transforming potential at each birth that reminds me of the imagery offered by De Chardin (1955/2003) in how who we connect and build upon history like

> ... a trunk that plunges down into the abyss of an unfathomable past, and whose branches rise somewhere ahead in a future, that at first sight, seems boundless. From this new perspective, the world appears to be a mass in process of transformation.

(16)

Likewise, birth brings new beginnings with silent blessings from the past that steer towards futures yet to be. A birth poem by S. Bowen (1992) aptly foregrounds this quality:

> ... from eternity to infinity.
> The cycle repeats itself,
> and the mystery remains.

(Cited in Hunter, 2000: 5)

The beauty of the past and future meeting in the present is at that moment an anticipation of the future and how that will unfold through the present time of birth. We are never confined to the present but always projecting towards the future from our pasts. This not a lineal progression of time, nor any other mode of movement such as spiralling or cyclic or repeatable; this is time when all notions of time converge in a felt moment. The Kairos moment of time at birth is a shared experience that finds us unexpectedly confronted by this enigmatic mystery, as Heidegger (1992) states: "The Now is not the momentary now of time, the *nunc fluens* but is the eternal now, the *nunc stans*" (45).

In the pursuit of change, reaching out, and grasping we move from one time to another creating a drive that propels us forward giving myriad perspectives on the world. As Heidegger argues it is this drive that allows for temporal succession. Yet the feeling of repeating cycles or moving from past to present to future are revealed in Kairos time in an eternal now. In Kairos time we are at once confronted with all of time without succession. This is an eternal now that invokes a profound intuitive leap into a depth of knowing gifted in that timeless mysterious moment. In this moment we glimpse divine vision and feel time conflated; Heidegger describes this eloquently as "... a single stroke without succession... God's present intuition reaches into the totality of time and into all beings that are in any time" (ibid.: 45).

Kairos and numinous experiences

Attuning at birth is how we converge with the totality of birth's interconnected experience. A unifying experience which lies hidden in the background awakens the spiritual significance of birth as a sacrament and proof of divine presence. A feeling of spiritual otherness or numinousness is a common aspect of being-there in that moment. There is gathering of others; seen and unseen, ancestors, and those yet to come disclosed by joy's awakening in that moment. It is plausible that numinous experiences at birth reveal personally transformative being-with-others at birth. Whoever and whatever this company of others may be, something in the experience is imminent, overwhelming and tangible, even sacred and holy.

This sense of 'sacred' and 'holy' can be construed as symbolic aspects of religious experience (MacKenna, 2009) that has coalesced from effective historical consciousness (Gadamer, 1960/1975). Whatever interpretation we bring to these words, the holy can be construed as something greater than us. The holy is named differently by different people. The word holy can inspire but can also be frustrating because it is invisible, immeasurable, and dependent on belief and/or faith. Yet humans are hermeneutic beings and all voices contribute to the meaning of holy. It is in the naming of things human beings are able to appropriate their experiences and give them meaning in the world in which we find ourselves. The birth experience uncovers a drawing near of divinity that puts us face to face with Rudolf Otto's holy-other as Dionysus the ecstatic liberator from worldly concerns "... something that captivates and transports ... with a strange ravishment, rising often enough to the pitch of dizzy intoxication..." (1917/1923: 31).

I am reminded of the lovely madness just after many births when everyone is intoxicated, fascinated, and enchanted. Something enchanting is experienced that can be a moment of transformation; a moment in which we find ourselves able to go forward into new understandings. Numinous encounters at birth set us free as we become overwhelmed "before the awe-inspiring" (ibid.: 17).

> As soon as baby came the father held his son up to the night sky offering an Islamic prayer, all the hairs on the back of my neck stood up. This was a holy moment, I continued to attend to the mother yet there was such a presence that touched and thrilled me to tears.
>
> (Personal field notes taken from my own midwifery practice)

Numinous experiences speak of the holy, reminding us of our love for life and the hope of new tomorrows. There is an unseen thread of life's love holding all together on an amazing journey of evolution. Others have appreciated how life begets life as an ultimate creative act (e.g. Arendt, 1958; Bergson, 1998/1911). There is something special at birth that draws close an intimacy with creation in Kairos time and numinous experience. This is also an embodied time reaching out and forming sacred space in all physical places, a time when seen and unseen, far and near, in clock time and beyond clock time, gather. This is a time when our world lights up suddenly, revealing a wholeness which penetrates deeply into our knowing of life bringing remembrance of what has always been there but taken-for-granted.

Like Klassen's (2001) claim that birth is a potent sacred state of spiritual significance, these non-rational aspects of maternity do not oppose the rational critical-thinking and decision-making often required at birth. On the contrary they have been understood as an expansion of such thinking (Parratt and Fahy, 2008). The non-rational aspects are part of being at birth, yet they are seldom acknowledged. Bringing the ineffable to speech without using notions that separate or dichotomise is the eternal challenge in western contexts. An underlying unity reveals something of significance common to the experience of being there at the time of birth. Even if not normally spoken, joy at birth opens a clearing to deeper knowing revealing something whole, non-fragmented, and profoundly meaningful about our shared fundamental human experiences of being alive.

Kairos and sacred joy

Joy is a multifaceted co-existing phenomenon. The experience of joy at birth harbours a message, hinting possibility. From nothing and no-where something at birth arrives and awakens: "*When I see the baby is actually coming; then it is the wonder and the joy*" (Marie). As we allow ourselves to be attuned and receive joy's message, happiness and relief bubble up. Joy as messenger at birth touches us and stirs up emotions once all have traversed the journey of birth "*it is touchable and tangible; it stirs up this happiness*" (Tui). Joy brings illumination to the gathering at birth that thrills and excites "*When this baby was out there was that happiness in the room. I would say it's pretty universal*" (Carol).

Such unveiling at the time of birth reveals our finitude as natal beings. It is a hint of the infinite unknown that stretches out before birth. That Kairos moment brings us face to face with an enigmatic mystery at the centre of our being; from where and to where is our origin? Science may help us understand where and how we arrive physically but "… that we are here remains mysterious … invites question and frustrates our attempts to provide answers" (O'Byrne, 2010: 20) for a "… baby is a creature fresh from eternity" (O'Donohue, 2012: 29) and beyond our limits of understanding.

Joy at birth is a grounding attunement that transcends everydayness and reveals and announces the sacred quality of the occasion as "*a powerful sacred moment*" (Cathy). To be sacred is to be venerated and regarded with great respect and reverence "*Like having all your hands up in the air, it is to be witness to the wonder and experience that spark of preciousness in that moment*" (Amy).

The joy of our shared natality

Kairos time at birth is a conjoining of past, present, and future "*in that moment the essence of everything meeting*" (Anahera). To be attuned to our shared natality is to be "grounded in the present moment, supported by the past that is arriving and the openness of a future that is calling" (Todnes and Galvin, 2010: 4). According to Arendt (1958) and O'Byrne (2010) there is an unfolding shared natal possibility in that moment that brings constant new hope. A hope that brings joy into our experiences of being there at birth. A joy that is not to be controlled or consciously desired but is an invitation into a clearing that reveals our shared destiny.

Arendt speaks of natality as an innate human condition. Natality lays bare our nature which constantly unfolds new beginnings and discloses our ability to be beginners of something new (Arendt, 1958). A baby is both in time and beyond time. A baby brings possibility for newness, a life to be lived, an unfolding potential for actualising dreams yet to be dreamt and realised. A baby reminds us of our shared natality and the creativity of generations as they are born. Birth is a miracle that holds the potential to positively progress the world. We stand amongst a host of others as "*a company of spirits arrive at birth that do something magic*" (Tui). We are awed in reverence at each miracle in the form of a baby and enjoy "*a special feeling around birth*" (Karl) in Kairos time.

Kairos and embodied natality

Natality's joy is a collective embodied experience in Kairos time (see Box 8.2). We are not the centre of the birth phenomenon yet at the same time we are part and whole of the experience. The moment of birth is unable to be broken into parts. Those at birth are already part of the world of birth in relationships. To attune joyfully is to yield to the call back to interconnected wholeness and our shared history and commonality. I am arguing that the occasion is a sacrament, a confirmation of the holy "*an expression and sacrament of the present moment*"

Box 8.2 Qualities of shared natality and Kairos time

- Moment in time conjoining past, present, and future
- Profoundly historical yet out of history
- Time that gestures unknown beginnings
- Transformative time gesturing newness
- Time of shared knowing and meaning
- Shared embodied celebratory felt-time
- Time of potential, possibilities, and opportunities yet to unfold
- Feeling of fullness, interconnectedness, wholeness, and authentic being together
- Time connected to feelings of journeying and continuity traversing generations
- Time that gifts value to birth
- A miraculous evocative shared felt-time invoking meaningful insights about life

Source: adapted from Crowther *et al.*, 2015

(Marie). The moment of birth is a gesture making visible life's web of significance, a source of hope, and testament to life's unending creativity. To witness birth is to be inspired; it is *"a strong experience, like seeing creation" (Brenda)*. It is a moment filled with embodied gratitude *"The soft tears were thankfulness and gratitude to God"* (Karl). To be there is to be fascinated and *"absolutely intoxicated!"* (Tui). The past is always revealed by decisions in any moment opening possibilities into futures. Our being at birth attuned joyfully reminds us of our shared responsibility to a future that matters to us. In that moment of shared natality joy is embodied through our tears, smiles, gentle voices, and tender touching *"like having a smile all over your body that spreads and doesn't go away"* (Tui).

Natality joyously gathers

Birth is symbolic and self-evident of beginnings that are transformative. It is not just a baby being born but others are being reborn into new relationships. Birth invokes a gathering, makes community; draws us nearer and authenticates a truly being-with unlike most other experiences in life *"an opportunity for us to grow closer together"* (John). Joy is the messenger of unifying love given from beyond. The dictates of the One temporarily fade into unimportance as we share smiles and hugs, tears, and celebration when a new human being arrives amongst us bursting into a galaxy of hopes and dreams. Birth inspires shared tender encounters *"I am present at the birth of their baby; an event which is special to them and which is special to me as well. It is lovely to be part of birth"* (Carol). In our togetherness at that precious yet vulnerable moment we are spellbound by life's continuing magnificence.

Attuned to joy we are released from our fragmented everyday existence. The joy loosens the hold of the One and everyday distractions authenticating us *"when he was born, I was shocked out of my everyday experience and feeling"* (Karl). We are always dealing with the unity of the whole at birth even if we cannot comprehend the wholeness and only 'see it' *"in a shadowy way"*

(Heidegger, 2008: 99). Birth acts as a catalyst of transition from a world of 'me' and 'I' or me-world to an experience of 'us' or a we-world as we glimpse our authentic selves. When we are not preoccupied with ourselves and activities, the sense of this unity assails us. In both its absence and presence, joy points to what matters most.

Safeguarding and sheltering what matters most

This inquiry reveals that birth is sacred even in busy maternity units. In these institutions, actions taken to preserve and protect something that is held with respect and reverence are glimpsed amongst contemporary maternity service provision. Safeguarding the space of birth allows joy to awaken. By turning and attuning to joy, recognition of something of significance calls out to us silently in the habitual turbulence of modern maternity care. It is a call to shelter and safeguard something precious and vulnerable. To safeguard is to surface and reveal our shared natality. It is taking care of something treasured so that it continues to 'be'. To safeguard is to attune to possibility. It is a revelation of truth about our always-already interconnectedness with others. The sacredness of birth is too valuable to be disturbed by inappropriate or discordant ways of being: "*I stay quiet because it's sacred, it's a special time*" (Dianne). To safeguard is to ensure its continuance, keeping it safe from harm and damage. If we treat the moment of birth with carelessness and brutishness, we risk losing the rarity of the gift of that Kairos moment. To respond to the call is to open the way to safeguard joy. It is a call to preserve and take under our care.

Joy calls us to a threshold in which we can dwell in delight, where the invisible comes into known presence "*There is a joy seen in their eyes as they see their baby for the first time; I tend to sit back a bit*" (Marie). This call is a reminder of our shared natality, a reminder of how birth matters. To attune to this call at birth is to arrive into deeper knowing of our collective presence. Joy is natality's messenger. Joy at birth is the mood of natality as life begetting life gifts hope and possibilities of better tomorrows. The essence of everything coalesces at birth attuning us to our common natalness. Joy at birth nears the world of our shared natality by shining a light on the occasion.

This inquiry reveals how joy arrives and assails us at the moment of birth deeply touching us. Joy's message is treasured and timeless conveying our unified existence beyond institutional structures, discourses, and social and professional differences. Joy is the grounding attunement at birth that authenticates us, joy is natality's messenger beckoning our collective response. Joy allows for existential freedom from the dictates of the One so that we fully surrender to the splendour of simply being assailed by birth's shared mystery. Joy is thus a sacred call that continuously whispers in the corridors and rooms of our hospitals, birth centres, communities, homes, midwifery, and medical schools in and around the time of birth. When joy at birth awakens it must be treasured, sheltered, and safeguarded lest it be damaged and lost leaving us bereft of possibilities. Joy awaits our open arms of gratitude and acceptance and invites us into the non-rational and the non-ordinary of our lives. Joy at birth authenticates us, brings us home, and reminds us of life's mystery that brings hope of new tomorrows. To come home is "to come in out of the winter of alienation, self-division and exile" (O'Donohue, 2012: 112). For that moment, birth turns us towards passion for life itself and an intimate tender being-with-other.

The language for articulating spiritual birth experiences are essentially silenced until permission is given to speak about them. It is in the speaking that the phenomenon of joy at birth becomes manifest and is made visible. The speaking lets joy at birth show itself in discourse. Yet there is much that remains mysterious. There is something at birth for it is not possible for there to be nothing. The nothing is something hidden in the ineffable, unspoken, or unsayable experience of joy. Yet I am reassured that what remains ineffable can provide: "...peace that passes understanding, and of which the tongue can only stammer brokenly. Only from afar, by metaphors and analogies, do we come to apprehend what it is in itself, even so our notion is but inadequate and confused" (Otto, 1917/1923: 34).

Conclusion

Birth unfolds in Kairos time, a moment of ecstatic clarity and peak experience in which our shared natality is made known to us, by the arrival of joy. Joy assails us, intones, and turns us to peace. The experience of being there at that special moment is addictive, thrilling, and magnetic for those present. When we turn to joy at birth, we are able to come to know ourselves more and enjoy the ever-renewing unity of life's potential beyond our everyday concerns and the expectations of what the One dictates. The fragrance, sound, touches, and seeing at birth are both poetically immanent and transcendental. This is an embodied feeling that invokes a smile which spreads all over our body stirring up tears of joy. To attune to joy at birth is to be touched and honour the ultimate gesture of life's love of life. The lived-experience of attuning joyfully at birth hints at the heart of humanity's endless creativity leaving a trace of holy presence in our everyday lives. We are called upon to shelter and safeguard something ineffable in that treasured moment. For, in joy's awakening, a shared feeling presence draws near that reminds us of what matters most.

Note

1 Etymologically the word numinous is from the Latin word numen, meaning "divine will" or "nod". Often associated with experiences that are non-rational and non-sensory and whose primary object is outside oneself. However, Rudolf Otto contends that the numinous is always multifaceted and resists being defined in terms of other concepts or experiences because it can only be evoked and awakened. Otto describes the numinous as a feeling that by its

> ... *nature is such that it grips or stirs the human mind with this and that determinate affective state ... [it] may at times come sweeping like a gentle tide pervading the mind with a tranquil mood of deepest worship. It may pass over into a more set and lasting attitude of the soul, continuing, as it were, thrillingly vibrant and resonant, until at last it dies away and the soul resumes its 'profane', non-religious mood of everyday experience. It may burst in sudden eruption up from*

the depths of the soul ... [It] may become the hushed, trembling, and speechless humility of the creature in the presence of – whom or what? In the presence of that which is a Mystery inexpressible and above all creatures.

(1917/1923: 12–13)

References

Arendt, H. (1958). *The Human Condition*. Chicago, IL: University of Chicago Press.

Bergson, H. (1998/1911). *Creative Evolution*. New York: Dover.

Crowther, S., Smythe, L., and Spence, D. (2015). Kairos time at the moment of birth. *Midwifery*, 31, pp. 451–457.

De Chardin, P.T. (1955/2003). *The Human Phenomenon*. Brighton, UK: Sussex Academic Press.

Gadamer, H.G. (1960/1975). *Truth and Method*. New York: Seabury.

Heidegger, M. (1992). *The Metaphysical Foundations of Logic*. Bloomington, IN: Indiana University Press.

Heidegger, M. (2008). What is metaphysics? In: D.F. Krell, ed., *Basic Writings*. London: Harper Perennial Modern Thought, pp. 89–110.

Hunter, L.P. (2000). *BirthWork*. La Jolla, CA: Pacifica Editions.

Kazenshe, D. (2004). *Kairos Time*. Available at: www.faithwriters.com/article-details. php?id=11461.

Klassen, P.E. (2001). *Blessed Events: Religion and Homebirth in America*. Princeton, NJ: Princeton University Press.

MacKenna, C. (2009). From the numinous to the sacred. *Journal of Analytical Psychology*, 54, pp. 167–182.

O'Byrne, A. (2010). *Natality and Finitude*. Indianapolis, IN: Indiana University Press.

O'Donohue, J. (2012). *The Four Elements: Reflections on Nature*. London: Transworld Ireland.

Otto, R. (1917/1923). *The Idea of the Holy (Das Heilige)*. London: Oxford University Press.

Parratt, J. and Fahy K.M. (2008). Including the nonrational is sensible midwifery. *Women and Birth*, 21, pp. 37–42.

Todnes, L. and Galvin, K. (2010). 'Dwelling-mobility': An existential theory of well-being. *International Journal of Studies Health and Well-being*, 5444, pp. 1–6.

White, E. (1987). *Kaironomia: On the Will-to-Invent*. Ithaca, NY: Cornell University Press.

9 Thinking anew

This chapter draws together the preceding chapters and suggests meaning and significance of these insights about joy at birth. To begin, I revisit what has been understood so far and show how multiple horizons of understanding reveal the phenomenon joy at birth, personal and professional, the voices of study participants, and the horizon of other literature. This is only a brief survey of the published literature and does not intend to be comprehensive and simply highlights possible resonances with the insights surfaced with this inquiry.

The horizon of other literature

The topic and focus of this inquiry are especially pertinent after publication of the WHO intrapartum guidance (2018) which recommends, amongst many things, the need to focus on outcomes that are more than mother and infant survival. The WHO guidance on intrapartum care draws our attention to the need for all involved to also thrive and reach their full potential. Similarly, in health care provider research, specifically midwifery, the need to ensure emotional wellbeing, for example, by attuning to a joy of practice has been shown to help a sustainable midwifery workforce (Kirkham, 2011; McAra-Couper *et al.*, 2014). Although no other published or unpublished research specifically examined the joy at birth, some attuned proximally to the phenomenon even if the same depth was not there. My hermeneutic literature review found that most published research breaks birth into parts, investigating and reporting on defined aspects such as satisfaction with the birth experience, place of birth, type of birth, and type of maternity care provider. Yet none examined the existential aspects as one phenomenon: "joy at birth" (Crowther *et al.*, 2014a).

Being-with-others

This inquiry uncovered a recurrent theme of being-with-others that was part of joy at birth not shown before. Voices of others often silenced in the gathering at birth were invited into this research. For example, although obstetric medical voices would appear dominant in published literature, obstetricians' experiential understandings are largely absent. Yet instead of defining obstetricians as different to others at birth, the experiential shared commonness of the moment through difference is revealed. Other studies have explored the experience of fathers at birth, reporting adverse emotional responses as well as uplifting experiences (Dellman, 2004; Johansson *et al.*, 2012; Kunjappy-Clifton, 2007; Lahood, 2006; Premberg *et al.*, 2011; White, 2007). Further studies have shown birth's influence on others, for example, grandmothers (Taubman-Ben-Ari *et al.*, 2011; Ben Shlomo *et al.*, 2010).

The shared meaning of joy experienced by family and friends as well as health care providers remained privative in the literature. There was paucity of evidence about how intimate others attuned to each other, the environment, and professionals. I acknowledge that not all intimate others were included, such as same sex partners, non-gestational mothers, siblings, and friends. However, what has been revealed are the hidden meanings from the wholeness of the shared attuned experience for everyone there in ways not addressed previously. To be at birth is a unique opportunity that gestures interconnectedness to others and the environment. Although separate and unique, we are connected and together in common ground not shown previously in the literature. Joy at birth shines a light and reveals the concealed truth of this unity that crosses cultural, social, and gender differences.

Felt-space at birth

The way place and space of birth co-exist in dialectic flow of inseparable con-joined wholeness with others has been uncovered in this inquiry. Several studies have inferred a special atmosphere or tone at birth (e.g. Berg *et al.*, 2012; Ólafs-dóttir, 2009), yet the phenomenon had remained for the most part unexplored. What is evident is that the phenomenon joy at birth is often unaffected by local-ity but can be disturbed and turned away from by those in that space. There is a mood at birth that opens a space within places that experience birth; this is a space that can be disrupted and treated in a brutish way and needs to be pro-tected (Crowther *et al.*, 2014b) lest the sacred quality of that space be undermined (Crowther, 2013).

Embodied joy

Intensity of embodied experience is integral to the experience as a whole. The meaning of embodied joy merges with others and reveals the wholeness of birth rich in meaning beyond that already articulated in the literature. The embodied nature of joy as revealed as shown in this inquiry is reflected in other studies (Dixon *et al.*, 2013a, 2013b). However, mention of joyful states relates to physi-ological changes for the mother and focuses on criteria measuring maternal satisfaction. The constitutive experiential aspects of joy at birth for all those present are not adequately described. Neither did measuring joy as part of satis-faction acknowledge the shared quality of joy at birth. Carter (2009) acknow-ledges embodied joy at birth as an incomprehensible connecting spiritual experience that facilitates integration with all aspects of life. How the integration for all who gather at birth is a new insight revealed in this inquiry.

Felt- time at birth

The lived-experience of non-clock time and felt time is constitutive of the joy at birth. Clock time as a lineal process of structuring and controlling birth has been explored previously (Downe and Dykes, 2009) but the timeless, special quality of that moment when a baby is born needed to be brought further into the light to appreciate its significance. Notions of intergenerational hope and future possibilities unfolding from a past into futures in this moment of birth have been revealed. For example, the philosophical notions of generation (Dilthey, 2002) and natality (Arendt, 1958; O'Byrne, 2010) have been reflected in this inquiry as central to the meaning of birth for everyone. The intergenerational experience at birth for birthing mothers has been highlighted elsewhere (Carter, 2009); yet this quality of felt-time has not been shown as shared experience previously. This quality of time is a time of growth and existential meaning (Taubman-Ben-Ari *et al.*, 2011). Naming this special time at birth as Kairos is a new and significant insight into spiritual experiences at birth and continues to be explored (Crowther *et al.*, 2015).

Spiritual experiences at birth

The different expressions of specialness in this inquiry point to a commonality of a unifying peak experiential moment that can be defined as spiritually mean-ingful. The interpretation of peak experience in this inquiry resonates with Maslow's (1964) peak experience as one in which there is a sudden joyful unify-ing phenomenon inducing spiritual feelings. The experience of joy at birth in this inquiry showed itself as such a peak experience. These birth peak experi-ences have been suggested in previous works, albeit they have not emphasised the unifying quality that Maslow suggested (Hoffman *et al.*, 2012; Schneider, 2012; Crowther and Hall, 2017; Lahood, 2007; Moloney and Gair, 2015). Peak spiritual experiences are shared at birth, even when not articulated and acknow-ledged. To be at birth affects us on some level; spiritual and existential experi-ences at birth gesture to something about how birth holds spiritual meaning and numinous mystery. Although these sacred qualities have been shown previously, much of this previous work across several disciplines has focused on individual experiences (Callister and Khalaf, 2010; Doherty, 2010; Etowa, 2012; Gray, 2011; Lennox, 2002; Linhares, 2012; Sered, 1991; Moloney and Gair, 2015), and not foregrounded how such sacredness can be felt by *all* there at the moment of birth when there is tact, sensitivity, and a turning towards joy.

Meaning of joy

Joy is a multifaceted co-existing phenomenon. Joy as a gathering and shared phenomenon at birth harbouring hidden meanings has not previously been explored in depth. This inquiry offers a rich phenomenological description and hermeneutic interpretation of that lived-experience across professional roles, dif-fering points of view, types and place of birth in ways not attempted by other researchers. Much of what is published about joy at birth in the literature conveys a clichéd entanglement of differing or opposing points of view (Crowther *et al.*, 2014a). Joy at birth is a phenomenon that is always partly in shadow, always partly withdrawn. This inquiry, from its genesis, attuned to an ontological inquiry and belies any notion of fixed characteristics. Revealing of the phenomenon joy at birth is always going to be a work on the way. Foregrounding the significance and meaning of joy at birth invites us to consider what the implications are. Likewise, the importance of experience of childbirth from multiple experiential and theoretical perspectives needs to be part of any recommendations.

Implications and recommendations

Joy has special meaning for all who are present at birth. There are common meanings that allow for difference in differing circumstances that highlights how being at birth is a shared experience which touches everyone. Therefore, any implications and recommendations arising from this inquiry cannot be solely directed at one social or professional group. In addition, those in physical proximity to birth, as well as those who are not close physically, need considering as they are all collectively part of a natal society.

Proximity at birth

This inquiry is a call to foster gentleness, tenderness, and humility at the moment of birth. This is a call to attune to a moment of sacred, quiet awe that invokes reverence and unobtrusiveness regardless of our role or relationship to the birth. Even in busy maternity care we can be humbled by mystery in which all concerns and distractions fall away as we attune to that moment of joy. There is a glimpse of something more pervasive than the professional and personal challenges of birth alone. Birth is an existential transformative and uplifting experience that has for the most part been hidden and forgotten. Yet there is a common feeling that points to something extraordinary that calls us to 'let the guard down'. There is a moment of grace that desires us to come together in a dance of stepping in and stepping back within joy's power; a moment that belongs to the family yet belongs simultaneously to all beyond the confines of the physical 'place' where the birth happens.

Turbulent moods as birth approaches have been revealed as constitutive of the childbirth experience in this study yet such changing affective states tell us little of the shared ontological attunement at the actual moment of birth. This inquiry reveals that there is an overwhelming existential wonder at that moment of birth which may feel out of control but still feel joyful despite seemingly adverse circumstances. To be uplifted and joyful at birth is a common theme through the experiences of those present.

Has the 'good birth' been construed as birth in the absence of interventions that are either required or requested? Has achieving a normal physiological birth been the apogee of a good birth? The notion of the 'good birth' concerns so much more than perhaps first understood (Smythe *et al.*, 2016). This inquiry reveals that birth is something far more profoundly significant and uplifting, hinting at experience beyond that commonly understood. This is not to generalise and assume that circumstances of labour and birthing can be distressing for some, for indeed, it can be. There are times when birth is experienced as dread and misery. In times of breakdown at birth when things go wrong, joy remains hidden. Yet this does not diminish the mystery and wonder of birth. What this insight is pointing to is the time of birth is always in some way a meaningful experience. For example, the homebirth and the forceps birth both gifted moments of joy in the participant accounts. Whether joy arrives and assails everyone in all other situations remains unknown.

The insights of this inquiry are a message of hope for those who find themselves completely positioned in technology or trauma who may feel they are bereft of meaningful experiences and unable to attune joyfully at birth. It is also a message of solace for those not physically present in those precious moments: the mother under general anaesthetic for caesarean section, for example, or the grandfather hearing news of a new grandson on his voicemail after the event. This is a sacred moment of human experience that attunes joyfully; a joy that cannot be manufactured for it arrives when the time is right. However, and wherever a baby is born it is always significant and meaningful. Even in a high-risk situation when joy is delayed, it can be anticipated and welcomed. This can be conveyed to families, explored by health care providers, and emphasised through media and social networking online sites.

Remember that the time of birth is *always* significant.
That moment needs to be sheltered and safeguarded in *every* circumstance.

To remember that moment's vulnerable yet powerful 'now' is to shelter and safeguard it. This inquiry calls us to reclaim something special at birth by sheltering the joyous experience and bringing it to voice. To name joy at birth is to presence and safeguard its possibility, as Heidegger (1971/2001) reminds us, "To save really means to set something free into its own presencing" (150). It is for those present at birth to be there in a sensitive way; attuned to holding sacred space. Sensitivity at birth frees joy into its own presencing. This points to the notion of holding safe space in midwifery (Taylor, 2010).

Taylor argues that the midwife acts as a container holding the boundaries of this safe space. Kirkham (2011) cautions that fearful space makes birth unsafe and as such trust is needed. Holding a safe space that is unthreatening and full of trust shelters and allows joy to awaken and helps the space to become sacred (Lemay and Hastie, 2017). Safe space is therefore an attribute of sacred space and is a call to everyone there at birth to act skilfully. To hold the safe space at birth is to provide an opportunity to turn towards and attune joyfully and feel the fullness of our Being. For this is a sacred space in Kairos time. To hold this sacred space is to respect, surrender, accept, shelter with tenderness and compassion supporting the unveiling of something significant in our lives. Holding sacred space is to keep the moment in reverence and tenderness; to shelter, protect, and safeguard something of worth and importance with humility (Crowther, 2013). It is to resonate in a way that brings harmony.

Being present means sharing joy at birth and appreciating the simplicity of Being-with (Merleau-Ponty, 1962/2002). Co-experience and reciprocal relationships open us to moving beyond our conversations inviting us into more profound ways of attuning with one another that reveals our individual and collective presence. We touch others as they touch us. This is sheltering the Kairos time at birth, an opening of sacred space when new life arrives amongst us joining seen and unseen realms. A time of attuned joy that thrills and brings us home.

Yet what do we sometimes see? Are there times when idle chatter, clearing equipment, or using a mobile phone disrupt that special moment? Changing of shifts, knocking on the door and entry of unknown others would all seem discordant with this precious time. Midwives, for example, can have a great effect on the space at birth. Evidence suggests that midwives dashing and rushing in and out creates an atmosphere that lacks calm (Huber and Sandall, 2009). Many families, midwives, and obstetricians already know that birth is profoundly significant and meaningful, yet they can act insensitively at this precious time. Størksen *et al.* (2013) reported how previous subjective negative birth experiences have greater influence over perception of the experience than obstetric interventions and fear of birth alone. The majority of women in their study, who experienced interventions, did not report overall lack of satisfaction with the birth. There are often assumptions that traumatic births decrease satisfaction. Yet Harris and Ayers (2012) concluded that focus on the hot spots in birth care such as interpersonal difficulties, providing support and reassurance lessens traumatically experienced births. Seemingly it would appear that care-giver support and attitude contribute to increased satisfaction more than the amount of interventions used. The experience of care is important.

Health care providers need to pay closer attention to times when something special is revealed at birth, when there is the "celebratory over the clinical ... nature over the supremacy of technology" (Cheyney, 2011: 535 and 537). The challenge is to ask whether our actions at birth are sensitive, tender, and respectfully performed honouring that moment. Do we really need to disrupt that moment with routines and mundane concerns? This inquiry has highlighted the importance of allowing the moment to present in its fullness and reveals how stillness and silence encourage the essence of the shared experience to surface. The time of birth brings us to authenticity. It requires us to be mindful of how we attune and the importance of the mood we bring into the birthing space. The occasion should not to be hurried and rushed for fiscal or managerial reasons. It is Kairos time; a moment to pause and be savoured; a moment to feel touched and be awed.

Implications for natal society

Arguably, with reduced maternal and perinatal mortality rates in western society, for the first time in history we can afford to examine what it means to be born without fear of death. Contemporary birth culture, for the most part, has become so entangled with risk avoidance strategies that it is in peril of being diminished by excessive risk averse practices that make birth impersonal, clinical, and empty experiences. I would contend that allowing deeply meaningful felt experiences at birth to be buried under such dominate birth culture is a travesty. Now is the time to re-evaluate society's shared meaning of birth and how society attunes at birth.

Tania McIntosh (2012) contends that how a society interprets birth is fundamental to how a society functions. Cultural awareness and willingness to listen to the silenced voices that beckon sacredness at birth can be heard throughout human history. Authoritative obstetric and indeterminate (intuitive and felt) knowledge are both part of contemporary birth yet meet in an uneasy co-existence. Birth technology may reveal lifesaving opportunities for birthing women and babies but sole focus on these technologies can also risk concealing things of importance and lead to interpreting birth as fundamentally risky and fearful.

Advances in technology could threaten society's experience of the sacredness of birth by stripping it of meaning. This inquiry exonerates the voices of those who have had the courage to continue noticing and celebrating the sacred at birth. My plea is for health professionals to be surprised by birth so that we do not practice in ways that limit how and what birth 'is' to technocratic interpretations. Bergum (2007) claims that technology causes fragmentation by disturbing and disrupting the relational quality at birth. I would suggest that it is our *relationship* with technology at birth that needs addressing not the technology itself. I am not arguing that interventions are all bad or all good. It can be argued that interventions have a role to play to avert tragedy and allow joy to awaken. In situations in which intervention are not judiciously applied, joy can be hidden leading to misery and trauma. Indeed, leaping in too soon and applying over-zealous interventions is just as harmful as not leaping in quickly enough to avoid harm and poor outcomes denying a new family's possibilities. I would contend that to be at birth with reverence would alter our relationship to technology and with each other. Conversely, juxtaposing joy and technology is a false dichotomy. Technology should not be telling us what birth 'is' but assisting us to hold birth safely when required, allowing joy's awakening and sacred meanings to surface.

Our understanding is growing about how environment and what we do around birth impacts newborns (Ragusa *et al.*, 2019; Dahlen *et al.*, 2013; Odent, 2011). Furthermore, how society attunes at birth may affect the way we connect with each other and our ability to love. The growing impetus to implement midwifery continuity and models of care which enable relationships to be fostered over the childbirth year and how such a relational focus brings further safety, better outcomes, improved satisfaction for women and families, and more joy of practice for midwives is both interesting and thought-provoking (Homer *et al.*, 2019). Yet the relational aspect of birth reflects not just the connection between mother and baby, health care professional, and woman, it is all of these together as well as a felt connectedness to the environment. It is encouraging that emerging childbirth evidence across a range of disciplines show that environment – physical and psychosocial – and relationships are important (Downe and Byrom, 2019).

Physiology, spirit, and how we attune are starting to unify in science and the implications of this are a call to acknowledge that birth is more than the focus on material intervention and birth locations alone. The spiritual wellbeing of the baby being born also needs to be considered (Heidari *et al.*, 2015; Hall, 2017). Stanistav Grof (1985), a psychiatrist, suggested that traumatic and positive experiences around our own births have consequences for our lifelong development and spiritual awakening which affect the quality of our contributions to society. If Grof's assertion is correct, then there is a need to attend to the wholeness of birth; including the spiritual wellbeing of a baby birthing into our world. Birth begins an embodied relational connection that continues to unfurl into childhood (Wynn, 2002) and nature and nurture in some way both contribute to the infant's ongoing spiritual development (Gellel, 2019). Our physiological and emotional birthing make-up may now be in jeopardy of being transformed, steering us towards unknown evolutionary consequences that shape our continuing shared natal expression if we do not address this wholeness. The final words of Jean Liedloff's (1977) germinal text *The Continuum Concept* resonates today:

> Once we fully recognise the consequences of our treatment of babies, children, one another and ourselves, and learn to respect the real character of our species, we cannot fail to discover a great deal more of our potential for joy.
>
> (159)

Implications for medical and midwifery education

There is something significantly awe inspiring, non-rational, and immanent in the experience of joy at birth. Some health care providers remember, shelter, and safeguard the moment of birth even though they may work within a system that does not necessarily acknowledge or value this. Yet joy at birth has been shown to be forgiving (remember how Tui forgives the rushed midwife caring for her daughter and how Amy forgives the doctor who hurt her in the forceps delivery). In addition, exposing joy at birth and surfacing common meanings hold possibility to breakdown professional and ideological conflict as I have experienced whilst doing this inquiry.

My concern is that the lived-experience of attuning to joy and its layers of meaning at birth is rarely part of the student learning experience. Midwifery educational curricula are often laden with learning outcomes associated with getting to grips with modern technologies and medical advances. Having spirituality in the curriculum is challenging yet important and requires a different creative pedagogical approach (Mitchell and Hall, 2007). For example, Chandramohan's (2014) South African study found that nursing students exposed to spiritual content in their learning were better equipped to provide spiritual orientated care. Furthermore, given that the phenomenon 'joy at birth' dwells within lived-experiences, pedagogical approaches that enhance learning and appreciation of birth as special and significant by honouring these lived-experiences is essential. Andrea Gilkison's (2013) study found that when New Zealand midwifery teachers and students interpret narratives together there was a learning opportunity that led to greater experiential understandings of child-birth. This could include the experiential significance and meaningfulness of joy at birth. Gilkison found that the emotional involvement encouraged under-standing of otherness of the other in ways not possible through didactic approaches to learning. Narrative pedagogy would be a valuable addition to educational programs for obstetricians too. One to one tutorials and student focus groups provide further opportunities to develop beyond the tasks and objective material that often dominates assessment orientated midwifery and medical curricula.

For example, open questions elicit more than the physiological and bio-medical aspects: *"Tell me about the last birth you were at?"* A host of details may follow about who did what and how. Follow up questioning could be: *"Tell me about that moment when the baby was born? How was that moment different? Why did you turn the lights down?"* In this way students would be encouraged to ponder their actions and those of others at birth. Such an approach provides opportunity for exploring deeper knowing. Returning to essential meaning and felt experiences at the moment of birth also provides an avenue for debriefing students who have had exposure to difficult learning experiences in practice.

Greater exposure to the humanities within a science practice focused degree would enhance appreciation and seeing of the other. Opportunity to explore the arts, philosophy, anthropology, literature, social history, comparative religious studies, and spirituality would open and develop an appreciation of the invisible and less measurable dimensions of birth. What I am arguing for is a re-attunement to the way undergraduate midwifery and medical education is delivered. Using art and crafts to reveal significance and meaning around birth has already been shown to be educationally useful in midwifery (Davies, 2007; Hall, 2012). Similarly, midwifery and medical postgraduate studies should incorporate deeper philosophical discussion about birth. This would in time lead to a tone of contemplative thought on the nature of maternity work across disciplines. It would open potential for professional dialogues and collaborative research possibilities relating to ways of being and the shared nature of the birth experience.

The belief that this would be inefficient use of resources needs to be chal-lenged. I argue that the moment at birth cannot be bought. To treat it as such is to view it as a commodity that would cheapen what is gifted to us in that moment and lessen it. The moment of joy at birth holds value beyond fiscally motivated maternity services and educational institutions. Returning to what is often now deemed unnecessary content in health care professional academia would humanise and sensitise students, allowing trust and altruism to flourish (Zak, 2012). Aca-demia without philosophical underpinnings leaves university education privative of something essential (Rolfe, 2013). In this broadened educative approach, the person is not merely trained to perform a professional role but be better educated to appreciate and articulate the shared lived-experiences at birth. This is more than merely asking questions about spiritual and religious beliefs, faiths, and cultures in a formulaic way in an attempt to practice in culturally safe ways; this is about honouring human experience (Crowther and Hall, 2015).

Thinking further into possibilities

Hermeneutic phenomenological inquiry is both description and interpretation. It is a process of inquiry that foregrounds meaning and significance of lived-experiences. It is a way of understanding our shared world beyond absolute significations, previous conceptions, and labels; it is thus always an open-ended inquiry. A hermeneutic phenomenological inquiry is never truly complete and final. How could it be? We cannot flick a switch and stop thinking about something that has impassioned us. There is often a calendar date in which a research project ends, when a 'thesis' is submitted and examined yet the thinking continues. As Heidegger reminds us, entering the hermeneutic circle of any inquiry in the right way is important and challenging. However, what is not required is to get out of the circle and stop pondering! This inquiry leads us into the circle of ongoing contemplative thinking about birth. We can press pause to complete and meet examination and publication deadlines, but it does not mark the end of an inquiry.

The next and final chapter of this monograph expands upon my original PhD conclusions in 2013 and develops the notion of the ecology of birth that has been published previously (Crowther, 2017) and extended further in my reflective writings (Wojtkowiak and Crowther, 2018; Crowther, 2019) and those of others (De Labrusse *et al.*, 2018).

References

Arendt, H. (1958). *The Human Condition*. Chicago, IL: University of Chicago Press.

Ben Shlomo, S., Taubman-Ben-Ari, O., Findler, L., Sivan, E., and Dolizki, M. (2010). Becoming a grandmother: Maternal grandmothers' mental health, loss, and growth. *Social Work Research*, pp. 45–57.

Berg, M., Ólafsdóttir, O.A., and Lundgren, I. (2012). A midwifery model of woman-centred childbirth care – In Swedish and Icelandic settings. *Sexual and Reproductive Healthcare*, 3, pp. 79–87.

Bergum, V. (2007). Way of the mother. In: V. Bergum and J.V.D. Zalm, eds, *Motherlife: Studies of Mothering Experience*. Alberta, Canada: Pedagon Publishing, pp. 2–21.

Callister, L.C. and Khalaf, I. (2010). Spirituality in childbearing women. *The Journal of Perinatal Education*, 19, pp. 16–24.

Carter, S.K. (2009). Gender and childbearing experiences: Revisiting O'Brien's dialectics of reproduction. *NWSA Journal*, 21, pp. 121–143.

Chandramohan, S. (2014). *Spirituality and Spiritual Care amongst Professional Nurses at Public Hospitals in KwaZulu-Natal*. Unpublished: Faculty of Health Sciences, Durban University of Technology.

Cheyney, M. (2011). Reinscribing the birthing body: Homebirth as ritual performance. *Medical Anthropology Quarterly*, 25, pp. 519–542.

Crowther, S. (2013). Sacred space at the moment of birth. *The Practising Midwife*, pp. 21–23.

Crowther, S. (2017). Birth as sacred celebration. In: S. Crowther and J. Hall, eds, *Spirituality and Childbirth: Meaning and Care at the Start of Life*. London: Taylor & Francis, pp. 13–29.

Crowther, S. (2019). Birth and spirituality. In: Z. Laszlo and B. Flanagan, eds, *The Routledge International Handbook of Spirituality and Society*. London: Routledge, pp. 113–119.

Crowther, S. and Hall, J. (2015). Spirituality and spiritual care in and around childbirth. *Women and Birth*, 28, pp. 173–178.

Crowther, S. and Hall, J. (2017). *Spirituality and Childbirth: Meaning and Care at the Start of Life*. London: Taylor & Francis.

Crowther, S., Smythe, E., and Spence, D. (2014a). The joy at birth: An interpretive hermeneutic literature review. *Midwifery*, 30, pp. 157–165.

Crowther, S., Smythe, L., and Spence, D. (2014b). Mood and birth experience. *Women and Birth: Journal of the Australian College of Midwives*, 27, pp. 21–25.

Crowther, S., Smythe, L., and Spence, D. (2015). Kairos time at the moment of birth. *Midwifery*, 31, pp. 451–457.

Dahlen, H.G., Kennedy, H.P., Anderson, C.M., Bell, A.F., Clark, A., Foureur, M., Ohm, J.E., Shearman, A.M., Taylor, J.Y., Wright, M.L., and Downe, S. (2013). The EPIIC hypothesis: Intrapartum effects on the neonatal epigenome and consequent health outcomes. *Medical Hypotheses*, 80, pp. 656–662.

Davies, L. (2007). *The Art and Soul of Midwifery – Creativity in Practice, Education and Research*. London: Churchill and Livingstone Elsevier.

De Labrusse, C., Humphrey, T., Ramulate, S., and MacLennan, S. (2018). Delivering spirituality in maternity services: An example from two European countries. In: M. Delaporte and M. Martin, eds, *Sacred Inception: Reclaiming the Spirituality of Birth in the Modern World*. Lanham, MD: Lexington Books, pp. 151–166.

Dellman, T. (2004). 'The best moment of my life': A literature review of fathers' experience of childbirth. *Australian Midwifery Journal*, 17, pp. 20–26.

Dixon, L., Skinner, J., and Foureur, M. (2013a). The *emotional* and hormonal pathways of labour and birth: Integrating mind, body and behaviour. *New Zealand College of Midwives Journal*, 48, pp. 15–23.

Dixon, L., Skinner, J., and Foureur, M. (2013b). The emotional journey of labour – Women's perspectives of the experience of labour moving towards birth. *Midwifery*, 30(3), pp. 371–377.

Doherty, M.E. (2010). Voices of midwives: A tapestry of challenges and blessings. *The American Journal of Maternal/Child Nursing*, 35, pp. 96–101.

Downe, S., and Byrom, S. (2019). *Squaring the Circle: Normal Birth Research, Theory and Practice in a Technological Age*. London: Pinter & Martin Limited.

Downe, S. and Dykes, F. (2009). Counting time in pregnancy and labour. In: C. McCourt, ed., *Childbirth, Midwifery and Concepts of Time*. London: Berghaun Books.

Etowa, J.B. (2012). Becoming a mother: The meaning of childbirth for African-Canadian women. *Contemporary Nurse*, 41, pp. 28–40.

Gellel, A. (2019). Children and spirituality. In: Z. Laszlo and B. Flanagan, eds, *The Routledge International Handbook of Spirituality and Society*. London: Routledge, pp. 120–126.

Gilkison, A. (2013). Narrative pedagogy in midwifery education. *The Practising Midwife*, 16, pp. 12–14.

Gray, C. (2011). The woman's choice: Birth and the divine feminine. *Clinical Psychology*. Palo Alto, CA: Institute of Transpersonal Psychology.

Grof, S. (1985). *Beyond the Brain: Birth, Death, and Transcendence in Psychotherapy.* Albany, NY: SUNY Press.

Hall, J. (2012). *The Essence of the Art of a Midwife: Holistic, Multidimensional Meanings and Experiences Explored through Creative Inquiry.* Faculty of Arts, Creative Industries and Education, Bristol, University of the West of England.

Hall, J. (2017). Pregnancy and the unborn child. *Spirituality and Childbirth.* London: Routledge, pp. 73–85.

Harris, R., and Ayers, S. (2012). What makes labour and birth traumatic? A survey of intrapartum 'hotspots'. *Psychology and Health*, 27(10), pp. 1166–1177.

Heidari, T., Ziaei, S., Ahmadi, F., Mohammadi, E., and Hall, J. (2015). Maternal experiences of their unborn child's spiritual care: Patterns of abstinence in Iran. *Journal of Holistic Nursing*, 33, pp. 146–158.

Heidegger, M. (1971/2001). *Poetry, Language, Thought.* New York: HarperCollins.

Hoffman, E., Kaneshiro, S., and Compton, W.C. (2012). Peak-experiences among Americans in midlife. *Journal of Humanistic Psychology*, 52, pp. 479–503.

Homer, C., Brodie, P., Sandall, J., and Levy, N. (2019). *Midwifery Continuity of Care: A Practical Guide.* London: Elsevier.

Huber, U.S. and Sandall, J. (2009). A Qualitative Exploration of the Creation of Calm in a Continuity of Carer Model of Maternity Care in London. *Midwifery*, 25, pp. 613–621.

Johansson, M., Rubertsson, C., Rådestad, I., and Hildingsson, I. (2012). Childbirth – An emotionally demanding experience for fathers. *Sexual & Reproductive Healthcare*, 3, pp. 11–20.

Kirkham, M. (2011). Sustained by joy: The potential of flow experience for midwives and mothers. In: L. Davies and R. Daellenbach, eds, *Sustainability, Midwifery and Birth.* London: Routledge, pp. 87–100.

Kunjappy-Clifton, A. (2007). And father came too … A study exploring the role of first-time fathers during the birth process and to explore the meaning of the experience for these men. *MIDIRS Midwifery Digest*, 17, pp. 507–512.

Lahood, G. (2006). *Bearing in Mind: Birth, Fathers, Ritual And 'Reproductive Consciousness' in Transpersonal Anthropological Perspective.* PhD thesis, Massey University, Auckland, New Zealand.

Lahood, G. (2007). Rumour of angels and heavenly midwives: Anthropology of transpersonal events and childbirth. *Women and Birth*, 20, pp. 3–10.

Lemay, C. and Hastie, C.J. (2017). Holding sacred space in labour and birth. In: S. Crowther and J. Hall, eds, *Spirituality Childbirth: Meaning Care at the Start of Life.* New York: Routledge.

Lennox, S. (2002). *Honouring the Sacred in Childbirth; A Midwife's Stories of Women's Developing Sense of Self.* Wellington: Victoria University.

Liedloff, J. (1977). *The Continuum Concept: Allowing Human Nature to Work Successfully.* Reading, MA: Addison-Wesley.

Linhares C.H. (2012). The lived experiences of midwives with spirituality in childbirth: Mana from heaven. *Journal of Midwifery and Women's Health*, 57, pp. 165–171.

Maslow, A. (1964). *Religions, Values and Peak Experiences.* Columbus, OH: Ohio State University Press.

McAra-Couper, J., Gilkison, A., Crowther, S., Hunter, M., Hotchin, C., and Gunn, J. (2014). Partnership and reciprocity with women sustain lead maternity carer midwives in practice. *New Zealand College of Midwives Journal*, 49, pp. 27–31.

McIntosh, T. (2012). *A Social History of Maternity and Childbirth: Key Themes in Maternity Care.* London: Routledge.

Merleau-Ponty, M. (1962/2002). *The Phenomenology of Perception.* London: Routledge Classics.

Mitchell, M. and Hall, J. (2007). Teaching spirituality to student midwives: A creative approach. *Nurse Education in Practice*, 7, pp. 416–424.

Moloney, S. and Gair, S. (2015). Empathy and spiritual care in midwifery practice: Contributing to women's enhanced birth experiences. *Women Birth*, 28, pp. 323–328.

O'Byrne, A. (2010). *Natality and Finitude*. Indianapolis, IN: Indiana University Press.

Odent, M. (2011). *Primal Health Research Database*. Available at: www.primalhealthresearch.com/introduction.php.

Ólafsdóttir, Ó.A. (2009). Inner knowing and emotions in the midwife-woman relationship. In: B. Hunter and R. Deery, eds, *Emotions in Midwifery and Reproduction*. New York: Palgrave Macmillan, pp. 192–209.

Premberg, Å., Carlsson, G., Hellström, A.L., and Berg, M. (2011). First-time fathers' experiences of childbirth: A phenomenological study. *Midwifery*, 27, pp. 848–853.

Ragusa, A., Rugolotto, S., D'Avino, S., Incarnato, C., Meloni, A., and Svelato, A. (2019). Off to a good start: Environmental imprinting in the childbirth period. *Journal of Pediatric and Neonatal Individualized Medicine (JPNIM)*, 8, p. e080127.

Rolfe, G. (2013). Thinking as a subversive activity: Doing philosophy in the corporate university. *Nursing Philosophy*, 14, pp. 28–37.

Schneider, D.A. (2012). The miracle bearers: Narratives of birthing women and implications for spiritually informed social work practice. *Journal of Social Service Research*, 38, pp. 212–230.

Sered, S.S. (1991). Childbirth as a religious experience? Voices from an Israeli hospital. *Journal of Feminist Studies in Religion*, 7, pp. 7–18.

Smythe, E., Hunter, M., Gunn, J., Crowther, S., Couper, J.M., Wilson, S., and Payne, S. (2016). Midwifing the notion of a 'good' birth: A philosophical analysis. *Midwifery*, 37, pp. 25–31.

Størksen, H.T., Garthus-Niegel, S., Vangen, S., and Eberhard-Gran, M. (2013). The impact of previous birth experiences on maternal fear of childbirth. *Acta Obstetricia et Gynecologica Scandinavica*, 92(3), pp. 318–324.

Taubman-Ben-Ari, O., Shlomo, S.B., and Findler, L. (2011). Personal growth and meaning in life among first-time mothers and grandmothers. *Journal of Happiness Studies*, 13(5), pp. 801–820.

Taylor, M. (2010). Midwife as container. In: M. Kirkham, ed., *The Midwife–Mother Relationship*. London: Palgrave Macmillan Limited, pp. 232–249.

White, G. (2007). You cope by breaking down in private: Fathers and PTSD following childbirth. *British Journal of Midwifery*, 15, pp. 39–45.

WHO. (2018). WHO *Recommendations: Intrapartum Care for a Positive Childbirth Experience*. Geneva: World Health Organization.

Wojtkowiak, J. and Crowther, S. (2018). An existential and spiritual discussion about childbirth: Contrasting spirituality at the beginning and end of life. *Spirituality in Clinical Practice*, 5, pp. 261–272.

Wynn, F. (2002). The early relationship of mother and pre-infant: Merleau-Ponty and pregnancy. *Nursing Philosophy*, 3, pp. 4–14.

Zak, P.J. (2012). *The Moral Molecule: The Source of Love and Prosperity*. London: Bantam Press.

10 Ecology of birth

This chapter represents further thinking and writing since completing the formal phenomenological inquiry and includes ongoing development and thinking pertaining to an ecology of birth. Having shown joy at birth through this inquiry, this chapter leans more towards a theoretical piece of writing than previous chapters, evolving in response to my growing sense that purely prioritising atomised material aspects of childbirth impede our capacity to attune joyfully when a baby(s) is born. Moreover, I was worried the phenomenon of joy at birth would be overlooked in our busy fragmentary personal and professional lives. I wrote the following piece in my reflective diary after completing the inquiry and attending a birth in answer to this question: '*What is most alive in us at birth?*'

> Befriend your experience at birth
> Slow
> Pause
> Pour awareness into your experience
> Feel joy's touch
> allow your natural vulnerability surface
> Embrace the intense surge within and around you and open
> Let joy joy itself from itself
> see time-space-others conjoin
> meeting your embodied presence
> Encounter your own core tenderness,
> yield to its intimacy, warmth, kindness
> Accept the invitation for wholeness in that moment,
> let the fragmentary idea of the world melt away
> This is poetry of life –
>
> a spontaneous arrival of mystery in the everyday
> Emerging within our collective presence
> we are awed when addressed by our most magnificent act of creativity

Joy at birth beckons our response in this fragmentary world, stirring and arousing us with overwhelming magnificence and creativity that gifts us feelings of an enduring wholeness. Yet, often, aspects of childbirth are addressed separately (e.g. staffing, buildings, institutional cultures and models of care, professional perspectives, and family's spiritual orientation). This artificial separation leaves the whole to fend for itself in the hope that somehow the parts will coalesce into an effective and acceptable whole that flourishes and sustains. This approach denies the inter-relational world of childbirth and risks losing something precious that could surface if the whole and parts were understood together. I am not the first to be concerned about the current fragmentary approaches in childbirth care. Hammond and Foureur (2019) explore the interconnectivity in the birth room and propose a concept of interconnectivity to support normal birth. Their interpretation of interconnectivity encompasses a mutual exchange or influence between all the parts that make up childbirth and suggest four interconnected domains of influence in the birthing room: spatial, neurobiological, behavioural, and cultural. This body of work is a useful addition to the literature and signals the need to view what goes on in the birthing from a more holistic perspective. In particular they unpack how neurobiological processes are affected by the physical environment and how this influences the culture of institutions and how practitioners and families behave. They conclude:

> We argue that the design and aesthetics of any space have direct neurobiological effects on the users of the space, which in turn shape behaviour and this contributes to the construction and expression of culture in both the physical and discursive environment.

(188)

I could not agree more, yet their analysis is mainly concerned with ontic or material aspects, whereas my focus is on an ecology that speaks to the ontological experiences unfolding in the spaces around birth; specifically, how all the parts and the whole gather together in the birth room and attune to mood within a significant temporal experience. As Heidegger reminds us:

> A space is something that has been made room for, something that is cleared and free, namely with a boundary ... A Boundary is not that which stops but, as the Greeks recognised, the boundary is that from which something *begins its presencing.*[1]

(1971/2001: 152)

Neither Hammond and Foureur's work or mine, or indeed the thinking of others who also speak about these concerns, are right or wrong – it is not about this or that – it is about all of it together. Each horizon of understanding contributes to revealing what is presencing in the birth room.

As we ponder further the idea of ecology something begins to speak and surface a holistic non-reductionist interconnected wholeness. Ecology holds the possibility of opening us to possibilities of meaningful encounters and transformational experiences in which something begins to come into presence and awaken. An ecology of birth would thus acknowledge the other material measurable aspects without denying any one of them, because to deny or leave out any aspect risks losing something important in birth's relational wholeness. Indeed, attending to practices that facilitate physiological birth has been shown to enable transcendent birth experiences where maternity care models value physiologic birth (Kurz *et al.*, 2019). Moreover, a good or/and positive birth comprises many interconnected relational qualities (Smythe *et al.*, 2016). What I am speaking of here is how an ecological lens attempts to understand all the parts of an eco-system working together in a sustainable harmony.

Without doubt context is important and dynamic. Searle (2006) named an aspect of ontology 'social ontology'. This perspective understands our world as both constituting institutional facts (e.g. systems, processes, and models of maternity care) that are mutually agreed amongst us and non-institutional facts based on the laws of nature and the physical world. My intention here is not to fully explicate and critique social ontology, instead I use this notion as a way to draw attention to how birth is always relationally interconnected within and part of the contextual world in which it unfolds. As illustrated in Chapter 3, Context and Mood, birth has transitioned from a mood attuned to privacy, home, and intimacy to one of public gaze, institutions, and professional activity.

Western cultural practices around birth have moved from the social-spiritual and biological to mechanical. For example, mediaeval medicine would have viewed patients as part of an ecosystem, a community affected by subtle unseen entities, whereas today patient's[2] concerns are seen in isolation as part of a machine break-ing down; the unseen entities of today are bacteria and viruses (Yawar, 2019). Prior to this mechanical view of birth, attendants relied on observation and dialogue and less on the diagnostic technologies and standardised results. Birth has traversed industrialisation and embraced the technological age and now we are on the thresh-old of increasing artificial intelligence and machine learning – what these changes mean for birth is unclear. What is certain is that the social-political and cultural context will continue to evolve, and we need to be vigilant that nothing gets over-looked, ignored, lost or hidden in the policies and practices informing childbirth.

The restoration of balance in an ecosystem is not solely about fixing biological breakdowns through medical interventions; it is so much more. Materialistic values can focus us away from providing care that is spiritually orientated, compassionate, and sensitive lessening our personal and collective wellbeing and possibility for transformation. The risk of pursuing uniformity and a reductionist medical agenda is that birth becomes denuded of spiritual meaning and birth's ecological system becomes further out of balance. Only when recognition and honouring of all the parts can each part flourish and lead to an integrated wholeness of birth as it unfolds according to its uniqueness in and through time, place-space, and person(s).

A social ontology of birth signifies how birth is socially embedded and gestures to how we understand and bring meaning to birth, including religious, psycho-social, emotional, and spiritual meaning. In other words, we come to know birth as Dasein, openly engaged and embedded human beings in the world of birth and society. To reduce any one part and seek to understand it in isolation under a microscope in a laboratory type condition is not how we come to understand any-thing in its fullness. According to Anna Hennessey's (2018) analysis of birth's social ontology, any focus purely on the materiality (or ontic) aspects of birth risks overlooking the myriad implicit meanings. She explores how rituals, images, mental imagery, and childbirth objects are made significant by birth's social ontology and how these objects are full of interconnected and embodied meaning.

Although it is easy to comprehend birth as overflowing with meaning due to its social embeddedness, there are also further meanings arriving from a realm beyond what we commonly define as the social. Professional and lay birth attendants/partners all have some implicit understanding of what a human being is and how birth is meaningful, miraculous, and sacred, even if these are the words not used by them. Our being there at birth, in whatever capacity, is innately spiritual and profoundly relational whether we acknowledge that or not. A recent integrative literature review I conducted with colleagues highlighted this further. The review reveals how post-birth mental health may be associated with spiritual experiences in the birthing space, namely how the quality of relationships and kinship matter; how the significance of childbirth and spiritual experiences are important; how honouring spiritual growth and wellbeing is crucial, and how physical manifestations and embodied experiences around childbirth need acknowledging (Crowther, *et al.*, 2019). Although the review does not claim causations – more work is required for that – it does highlight the significance of how we are and how and what we do in birth space and time is important to birth ecology.

Arne Naess (1989), philosopher and environmentalist, coined the term 'deep ecology' that speaks of life's relational wholeness. The word 'deep' implies a depth of questioning into the fundamental causes of our concerns about natural systems, in this case, birthing the next generation. We therefore have a moral responsibility at each birth to be fully present and open to the gifts that such moments reveal. Naess tells us that awareness of problems is insufficient, and that wisdom is required to address what needs to be done. Likewise, we need to consider the impact of our actions and non-actions at birth for the sake of ourselves now and for generations to come. As part of this undertaking we must refocus and redesign our current maternity systems based on values and methods that safeguard joy at birth and all the elements of the ecology of birth that enable joy's awakening.

Joy at birth reveals itself through our experiential encounters, our fore-structures of understanding and how we bring meaning to events that we find ourselves thrown into. It shows us that we are always interested in the world in which we dwell and that is how we come to know what we know. What this inquiry has foregrounded is how birth provides us with meaning and purpose; it touches us all and is fundamental to who we are as it overflows with spiritual and existential significance that become named and understood by our social embeddedness. Yet, such meaning is often ineffable, resisting our attempts at naming and labelling that seek to confine our comprehension within our current horizon of understanding. The challenge of naming anything ineffable in our experiences is finding language that portrays a relational totality of human experience in its wholeness. Human beings have grappled with these questions for eons – unfortunately some of our questioning and subsequent actions have resulted in outcomes that may be lessening our view.

The ecology of birth (see Figure 10.1) represents a fusion of horizons informed by this phenomenological inquiry, a philosophical analysis of a good birth (Smythe *et al.*, 2016), Heidegger's four-fold structure of existence (Plebuch, 2010; Heidegger, 1971/2001) and my ongoing connection to the birthing world through research, postgraduate supervision, writing, education, policy and guideline development, and practice. What is consistently emphasised is that an ecology of birth is primordially about the interrelatedness of phenomena. The purpose of developing this ecological model is to draw our attention to a whole-ness regarding birth across all types of birth, wherever and however they happen, and what that means in the context of an ontological inquiry. Models can be problematic because they are often abstractions of things in the real world failing to fully reflect the richness and depth of lived experiences as lived in and lived through claiming some notion of generalisability. This would be incongruent with an ontological focus. So, I use this model with caution staying mindful not to imply a final conceptual schema of what joy is. That would be foolhardy and belie the ontological inquiry that forever remains open because it is impossible to fully unconceal any phenomenon.

This version of the ecology of birth model[3] has been extended through ongoing reflection and usage (see Figure 10.1). In addition to the four domains suggested by Hammond and Foureur (2019), this is made up of six overlapping and non-hierarchical areas surrounding the moment of birth. There is no hierarchy;

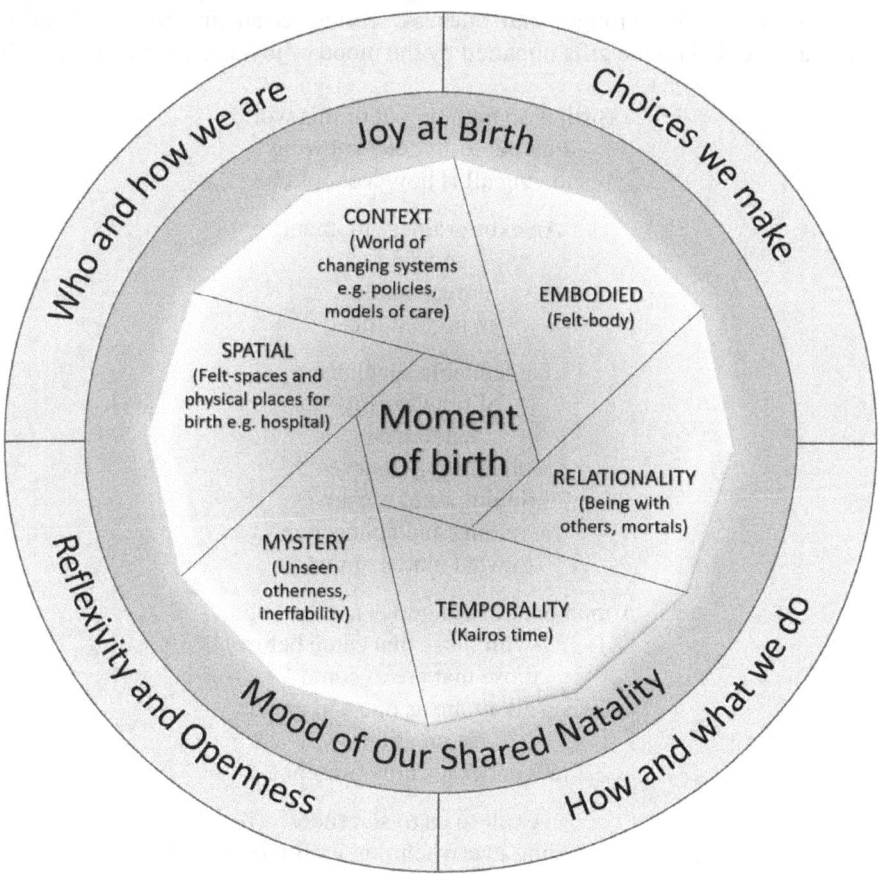

Figure 10.1 Ecology of birth.

each area dwells in the interiority of the other, weaving eternally within and between one another. What is added since the first iteration is how these six areas are constantly influencing the mood of our shared natality: joy. Further-more, the model now shows how joy is affected by us and by our choices in any given moment, namely, to turn towards or turn away from that joy, to work with or against joy in our actions, and how we are being. The ecology of birth high-lights how we need to remain open and engage fully with what we bring by adopting a reflexive stance. It also foregrounds how the environment affects our behaviour around birth. It signals how joy at birth touches us profoundly on many levels, for instance, as a felt embodied encounter experienced sensorially through touching, holding, smelling, seeing, and hearing along with visceral emotional affects such as weeping, smiling, and shaking.

How does this ecology of birth model show itself in experience? I return to the stories and poems of Chapter 7. The following poem uses the words of parti-cipants who gifted their stories to this inquiry. You have read their stories and brought them to your thoughts. They have become an emergent horizon of understanding within you – that is their gift. The following poem is a gathering of myriad insights brought into oneness serving as an invitation to hearing, seeing, and feeling the gifts imparted by the mood of joy at the moment of birth.

Birth is something out of this world
drawing forth deep knowing
showing all is how it should be

An extraordinary moment
amazing
unrepeatable
in normal life

Undefinable specialness
of timeless joy
tenderness
that deeply touches
bringing us to ourselves
reminding and connecting
to what matters most

A moment of beginnings and endings...
Being-with those that came before
those that are to come
when all attune as one and gather
in creation
in wonderous holy presence

A call to us to surrender
feeling overwhelming gratitude
we are stirred beyond words
right there in that moment

Personal call to action

Every birth includes a mysterious unspoken quality unfolding in and around the occasion; to honour that does not deny practice that keeps birth physically safe – but we must also keep birth emotionally and spiritually safe by safeguarding the meaningfulness of this human event. To focus purely on the biopsychosocial aspects of childbirth alone and ignore the spiritual aspect is unacceptable. In whatever way we approach birth, as woman/mother, educator, practitioner, researcher, chaplain, religious leader, writer, manager, health policy maker or politician, remember that birth is an ecology comprised of many aspects that all need acknowledging and safeguarding. We need post-materialist policy and management structures that enable deep ecology, trust, reciprocity, and relationships to flourish in our maternity organisations. Whoever we are, whatever role we take on around birth, whether we are directly involved, whether we are biological or non-biological parents or childfree, we are part of human society and are touched by birth somehow.

Current maternity systems are in crisis and often find us unable to be fully who we are because we are anxious about being ridiculed and being suddenly ripped away from the joy revealed in this inquiry. Yet, we can choose to lean into joy by being grateful for the role we have that allows us to be there and by being grateful for the moment of grace afforded in those precious moments. I'm reminded of Brené Brown's (2018) work on vulnerability when she encourages us to step up into our own power and be courageous. This phenomenological inquiry acts as a call to be brave and show up and change the status quo by moving beyond our comfort zone which requires us at times to be subversive. It is about choice and acknowledging what we bring to birth personally; it is about being courageous and facing the resistance we may encounter when we confront brutish actions and disempowering language around childbirth. This is an invitation to choose to feel any fear and discord around birth and respond proactively, in whatever capacity we are privileged to be there. My plea, when it seems fragmented and falling apart, become aware of how you may be allowing your lived experiences to cloud over with clutter and noise; in that moment re-attune to your embodied wisdom and allow your heart to break.

The alternative is to choose to be the cause of the fear and discord that exists in much of our contemporary birth culture. This requires us to be vulnerable and open ourselves to what is unfolding. Don't be afraid of drowning in the overwhelm of the moment when you open yourself up; I promise you can still breath when joy intoxicates you. We all have the capacity to transcend and participate in the sacred and seek connectedness, meaning, and purpose. Self-transcendence is about reaching beyond our everyday concerns and structures and engage fully with what fulfils us.

Joy is an invitation to reach and extend beyond ourselves. Joy can be understood as a form of relational spirituality and an opportunity to connect with the sacred at birth, generating an openness and cognitive flexibility which leads to thinking and acting anew. See, hear, and feel what is occurring inside and outside of you and allow yourself to be touched, brought to tears, and feel joy's gift of healing to wash over you when it arrives. The power of any gift is in its relational impact across time and space. To give and receive a gift is to forge a relationship, leaving a trace within each other of this mutual transaction. Like-wise, the gift of joy's arrival in the birthing room brings us into profound rela-tionship with life, leaving a trace of the ineffable in our lives whilst simultaneously bequeathing a trace of who we are in the seen, unseen, within, and between us of life's wholeness. As joy assails you at birth, you encounter an emergent relational connectivity embracing you and others which cultivates compassion that can be personally enriching. Stop telling yourself that you cannot do this and turn up completely in your humanness and be prepared to be vulnerable and open to modifying your worldview as a corollary of that experi-ence. This is about sharing our humanity in a celebration of life. The emergence of new life at each birth is its own ecology and it is all our responsibility to safeguard and shelter that which is most precious.

Closing thoughts

This inquiry calls us to think anew about birth and appreciate that all births are significant in all situations, whatever the outcome; whatever the social economic situation, place of birth, technology employed or type of care providers attend-ing. When we come together in a space of passion (like birth), something happens between us, yet often this 'thing' remains unnamed. This inquiry names this 'thing' joy. To be assailed by this joy at birth is an opportunity to be reminded of what matters most in and beyond the ordinary. My purpose is to guide us towards a greater acknowledgement of birth as something special by bringing that something to a feeling that foregrounds how birth is more than what is measurable, definable, more than what is within any research agenda, model of maternity care provision, and any discreet professional discipline juris-diction. It is about individuals and all of us together simultaneously. It is about the joy of being alive, a celebration of life, and depth of existential togetherness that brings our shared human experience into presence in that moment when a new life arrives amongst us. We don't simple birth because we have biological bodies – we birth each generation because we are creative Beings of ever new and unfolding possibilities. When we find ourselves present at the moment of birth, we are transformed by the mood of the moment as our own most creativity takes form. There is something about joy at birth that can inform our being there at birth and how we do what we do in those cherished moments. Hence, joy at birth is a phenomenon worthy of our ongoing concern and fascination.

Notes

1 Author's own emphasis in italics.
2 I prefer to use the words 'women' or 'woman' when speaking of childbirth care. Patient implies illness and a medical relationship with carers as opposed to a social model of care in which hierarchical relationships are transformed into partnerships.
3 See the original version in Crowther, S. (2017). Birth as sacred celebration. In: S. Crowther and J. Hall, eds, *Spirituality and Childbirth: Meaning and Care at the Start of Life*. London: Taylor & Francis, pp. 13–29.

References

Brown, B. (2018). *Dare to Lead: Brave Work, Tough Conversations, Whole Hearts.* London: Random House Publishing Group.

Crowther, S. (2017). Birth as sacred celebration. In: S. Crowther and J. Hall, eds, *Spirituality and Childbirth: Meaning and Care at the Start of Life.* London: Taylor & Francis, pp. 13–29.

Crowther, S., Stephen, A., and Hall, J. (2019). Association of psychosocial–spiritual experiences around childbirth and subsequent perinatal mental health outcomes: An integrated review. *Journal of Reproductive and Infant Psychology*, pp. 1–26.

Hammond, A. and Foureur, M. (2019). Interconnectivity in the birth room. In: S. Downe and S. Byrom, eds, *Squaring the Circle: Normal Birth Research, Theory and Practice in a Technological Age.* London: Pinter & Martin Limited, pp. 180–192.

Heidegger, M. (1971/2001). *Poetry, Language, Thought.* New York: HarperCollins.

Hennessey, A.M. and Davis-Floyd, R.E. (2018). *Imagery, Ritual, and Birth: Ontology between the Sacred and the Secular.* Lanham, MD: Lexington Books.

Kurz, E., Davis, D., and Browne, J. (2019). 'I felt like I could do anything!' Writing the phenomenon of 'transcendent birth' through autoethnography. *Midwifery*, 68, pp. 23–29.

Naess, A. (1989). From ecology to ecosophy, from science to wisdom. *World Futures: Journal of General Evolution*, 27, pp. 185–190.

Plebuch, D. (2010). *Heidegger's Fourfold.* Thesis. Graduate College University of Illinois, University of Illinois, Urbana.

Searle, J.R. (2006). Social ontology: Some basic principles. *Anthropological Theory*, 6, pp. 12–29.

Smythe, E., Hunter, M., Gunn, J., Crowther, S., Couper, J.M., Wilson, S., and Payne, D. (2016). Midwifing the notion of a 'good' birth: A philosophical analysis. *Midwifery*, 37, pp. 25–31.

Yawar, A. (2019). Spirituality in medicine. In: L. Zsolnai and B. Flanagan, eds, *The Routledge International Handbook of Spirituality in Society and the Professions.* London: Routledge, pp. 193–204.

Epilogue
Personal transformation

In the process of this inquiry I became acutely aware of the different cultural perspectives of others and how fusion of horizons of understanding occurs. The cultural conflicts between the natural and technocratic birthing cultures prevalent today in twenty-first century birthing practices echoed in the stories collected. There were dialectical descriptions of cultural identity within each paradigm, medical/technocratic, and natural/holistic/social. I found myself situated in the latter of these two worlds. I saw, in myself, how midwifery is constantly interpreting itself within its own discursive space. I saw clearly the internal divisions that constantly support and disprove aspects of my worldview. I was challenged by opposing interpretations. Lampert (1997) exhorts us to make familiar that which seems alien and conversely make alien that which seems familiar. In doing so, this inquiry has highlighted the distances and nearness between the cultures. Acknowledging that I am unable to 'put myself in others shoes' as Gadamer asserts (Gadamer, 1960/1975: 303–304), the importance of bringing these different voices to this interpretation allowed the diversity and commonality to surface.

All accounts of modern childbirth share a common ground and cultural history that harbors an excess of meanings to society. Lampert (1997) contends that through differences commonality is manifest. For example, I remember sitting in my car before an interview with a male obstetrician feeling nervous, believing that he would neither understand what I was doing nor agree with what I would find. Yet this was not the case and my interpretation of obstetricians and their world has transformed. As I came to appreciate our differences, our commonality manifested new insights. The differences in our traditions became understood more profoundly by the fusion of our interpretive horizons. The fundamental conflict that appeared to be evident in the two professional approaches to birth was essential to the interpretation of perspectives common to both. What had appeared alien became accessible on this journey. All professional groups self-interpret. My pre-understandings and those of the participants in this study were built by a history that was shared. It was such understanding that helped me recognise common concerns in the childbirth phenomenon. I now see that it is the common history of childbirth and its central importance to human society across traditions and history that provided the connecting point for mutual interpretation and deeper understanding.

Through bringing these differing perspectives to the interpretation, my horizons were brought into sharp relief, initiating questions about my own pre-understandings. Attempting to see the horizon of the other threatened what I held to be right in my own worldview of birth and thus helped me see facets of the phenomenon that had previously been hidden from me. At the start I found myself entrenched within a tradition to the exclusion of others. My sense of isolation from some practitioners and women who adhere vehemently to one approach to the exclusion of others paradoxically served as the very form of connectedness I sought.

I now appreciate how phenomena need to come to language for mutual understanding. Like the challenges in interpreting foreign words, words in our native tongue need to be challenged, clarified, and/or altered in order to under-stand the deeper meanings. I now listen to others, fascinated and intrigued by how in the act of listening interpretation changes as mutual understanding at the deepest level of human experience unfolds. The significance of this inquiry has forevermore informed my approach to practice, teaching, and research. The possibility of a common world of experience at birth has opened for me. The sacred call of joy whispers louder than before.

Hermeneutic phenomenological inquiry, when you surrender to its process, often initiates personal transformation. Whilst engaged in this inquiry I certainly experienced a remaking or evolution of my thinking, feeling, and appreciation of birth, both professionally and personally. I now see how spiritual conviction, belief or peak experience at birth has become a private affair. At the beginning of this journey I felt that there was a broken connection to the soul of birth. I now see that it is perhaps only in that special, even holy, moment at birth that something sacred and awe-inspiring touches us in ways that can mend the con-nection. As well as being transformed, there was a quality of transfiguration. Transfiguration in this context gestures to a revelation and perceived altered state about the underlining primordial nature of birth. The moments around birth had metamorphosed for me into something so much more than I had imagined. I became awestruck at the richness and felt I had encountered the holy within the stories of joy. During my inquiry I was asked 'What do you mean by holy?' This was my response at the time:

> Holy for me is something private, tender and special. It is a blend of western Christian theism and Asian mysticism. It is the profoundest rela-tionship in my life. It is an interconnecting knowing and loving, the source of all things; a creative force that provides and liberates. The Holy is invis-ible but whose actions are visible. It is the something ineffable, unexplaina-ble that peeps through a poem, a painting, a child's smile, the fragrance of an unfurling flower, the unseen artist painting the crimson dawn over the ocean. It is benevolent and seeks my happiness.
>
> The holy calls me to serve others as in that serving I feel closer to what is holy. It shows itself from its invisibility through my experiences. When I catch myself moved to tears by another, I know I have been touched by the holy. It is the glint in the eyes of all I meet every day and everywhere. It

shows itself in the 'simpleness' of being still and silent and in the raw of thunder and exploding volcanoes! When I stop and take notice the holy gazes back in the mirror. It is the wonder of body and senses. The holy holds all together and makes up the material of the physical earth; both immanent and transcendental.

The holy has a personality that attracts and inspires constantly sending messengers from beyond into my everyday life. It is all relationships in one. When I find myself in despair, I feel furthest yet the holy is nearer than my 'I'. The holy desires that I remember the deepest belonging and connection; the feeling that 'I am in love and loved'. I come to know the holy in special moments when the invisible touches and reminds me of who and what I am.

To be at birth is be close to the holy. To be a birthing woman, midwife or any other birth attendant and partner is to bear witness to the extraordinary in everyday life. My earnest wish is that a sense of the holy, whatever that is for you, has been awakened and inspires you to turn into joy at birth's call and feel its heartfelt welcome and healing embrace.

References

Gadamer, H.G. (1960/1975). *Truth and Method*. New York: Seabury.
Lampert, J. (1997). Gadamer and cross-cultural hermeneutics. *The Philosophical Forum*, XXVIII, pp. 351–368.

Index

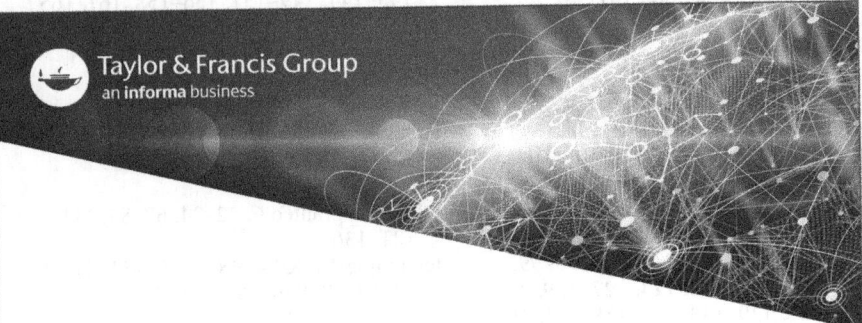
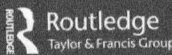
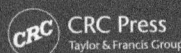